lueprints Q&A

PSYCHIATRY

D1614617

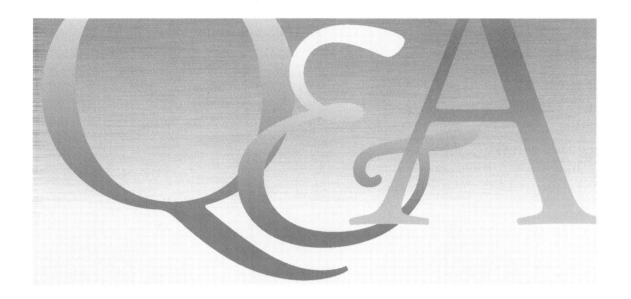

Blueprints Q&A
STEP 2: PSYCHIATRY

SERIES EDITOR:

Michael S. Clement, MD

Fellow, American Academy of Pediatrics
Mountain Park Health Center
Phoenix, Arizona
Clinical Lecturer in Family
and Community Medicine
University of Arizona College of Medicine
Consultant, Arizona Department
of Health Services

EDITOR:

James Brian McLoone, MD, FAPA

Clinical Professor in Psychiatry
University of Arizona
Chairman, Department of Psychiatry
Director, Residency Training
and Medical Student Clerkship
Good Samaritan Regional Medical Center
Phoenix, Arizona

LIBRARY
SWANSEA PSYCHIATRIC EDUCATION CENTRE
T CHURCH
CEFN COED HOSPITAL
COCKETT
SWANSEA SA2 0GH

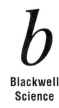

**Blackwell
Science**

©2002 by Blackwell Science, Inc.

EDITORIAL OFFICES:

Commerce Place, 350 Main Street,
    Malden, Massachusetts 02148, USA

Osney Mead, Oxford OX2 0EL, England

25 John Street, London WC1N 2BL, England

23 Ainslie Place, Edinburgh EH3 6AJ, Scotland

54 University Street, Carlton, Victoria 3053, Australia

OTHER EDITORIAL OFFICES:

Blackwell Wissenschafts-Verlag GmbH,
    Kurfürstendamm 57, 10707 Berlin, Germany

Blackwell Science KK, MG Kodenmacho Building,
    7-10 Kodenmacho Nihombashi, Chuo-ku,
    Tokyo 104, Japan

Iowa State University Press, A Blackwell Science Company,
    2121 S. State Avenue, Ames, Iowa 50014-8300, USA

DISTRIBUTORS:

The Americas
    Blackwell Publishing
    c/o AIDC
    P.O. Box 20
    50 Winter Sport Lane
    Williston, VT 05495-0020
    (Telephone orders: 800-216-2522;
    fax orders: 802-864-7626)

Australia Blackwell Science Pty, Ltd.
    54 University Street
    Carlton, Victoria 3053
    (Telephone orders: 03-9347-0300;
    fax orders: 03-9349-3016)

Outside The Americas and Australia
    Blackwell Science, Ltd.
    c/o Marston Book Services, Ltd., P.O. Box 269
    Abingdon, Oxon OX14 4YN, England
    (Telephone orders: 44-01235-465500;
    fax orders: 44-01235-465555)

Acquisitions: Beverly Copland

Development: Angela Gagliano

Production: Irene Herlihy

Manufacturing: Lisa Flanagan

Marketing Manager: Toni Fournier

Cover design by Hannus Design

Typeset by Software Services

Printed and bound by Courier-Stoughton

Printed in the United States of America

01 02 03 04 5 4 3 2 1

The Blackwell Science logo is a trade mark of Blackwell Science Ltd., registered at the United Kingdom Trade Marks Registry

Library of Congress Cataloging-in-Publication Data

Blueprints Q & A step 2. Psychiatry / editor,
James Brian McLoone.
    p. ; cm.—(Blueprints Q & A step 2 series)
    ISBN 0-632-04592-2 (pbk. : alk. paper)
    1. Psychiatry—Examinations, questions, etc.
    2. Physicians—Licenses—United States—Examinations—
Study guides.
    [DNLM: 1. Psychiatry—Examination Questions. WM 18.2
B658 2002] I. Title: Blueprints Q&A step 2. II. Title:
Psychiatry. III. McLoone, James Brian. IV. Title. V. Series.
    RC457 .B58 2002
    2001002138

Notice: The indications and dosages of all drugs in this book have been recommended in the medical literature and conform to the practices of the general community. The medications described and treatment prescriptions suggested do not necessarily have specific approval by the Food and Drug Administration for use in the diseases and dosages for which they are recommended. The package insert for each drug should be consulted for use and dosage as approved by the FDA. Because standards for usage change, it is advisable to keep abreast of revised recommendations, particularly those concerning new drugs.

CONTRIBUTORS:

Lori B. Highberger, MD
Resident in Internal Medicine and Psychiatry
Good Samaritan Regional Medical Center
Phoenix, Arizona

Lori received both her undergraduate degree in
Psychology in 1993, and her medical degree four
years later from the University of Kansas. She aspires
to one day open a geriatric medicine and psychiatry
clinic, while remaining involved in the teaching of
residents and medical students.

Patricia O. Kirby, MD
Resident in General Psychiatry
Good Samaritan Regional Medical Center
Phoenix, Arizona

Born in Ohio, Patricia attended The Ohio State
University College of Medicine. In 1992, an undergraduate degree was earned in Microbiology from
Miami University in Oxford, Ohio. Patricia now
specializes in the treatment of patients with eating
disorders. Her twin daughters Hope and Hannah
also lend to her active lifestyle.

James B. McLoone, MD, FAPA
Chairman, Department of Psychiatry
Director, Residency Training and Medical Student
Clerkship
Good Samaritan Regional Medical Center
Phoenix, Arizona

James received his medical degree in 1976 from
George Washington University School of Medicine in
Washington, DC. Attending the University of Arizona
for undergraduate study, he graduated in 1972 concentrating in both Zoology and Psychology. As a
third generation Arizonian, James was born and
reared in Phoenix. He thoroughly enjoys teaching
residents and medical students, but is most proud of
his two children Katie and Brian.

Jonathan Zuess, MD
Resident in General Psychiatry
Good Samaritan Regional Medical Center
Phoenix, Arizona

Jonathan received his medical degree in 1993 from
The University of Adelaide, in South Australia. He did
undergraduate work in Britain attending both a
naturopathic and homeopathic college. He is origi-
nally from Haifa, Israel. Jonathan is well published in
the field of Complementary and Alternative Medicine.

REVIEWERS:

M. Christian Cornelius, MD
Clinical Faculty Psychiatrist
Good Samaritan Regional Medical Center
Phoenix, Arizona

Marcelle D. Leet, MD
Vice Chair, Department of Psychiatry
  and Medical Director Inpatient Psychiatry Service
Good Samaritan Regional Medical Center
Assistant Clinical Professor of Psychiatry
University of Arizona College of Medicine
Phoenix, Arizona

Andrea J. Waxman, MD
Associate Director Education Programs
Department of Psychiatry
Good Samaritan Regional Medical Center
Phoenix, Arizona

PREFACE

The Blueprints Q&A Step 2 series has been developed to complement our core content *Blueprints* books. Each *Blueprints* Q&A Step 2 book (*Medicine, Pediatrics, Surgery, Psychiatry,* and *Obstetrics/ Gynecology*) was written by residents seeking to provide fourth-year medical students with the highest quality of practice USMLE questions.

Each book covers a single discipline, allowing you to use them during both rotation exams as well as for review prior to Boards. For each book, 100 review questions are presented that cover content typical to the Step 2 USMLE. The questions are divided into two groups of 50 in order to simulate the length of one block of questions on the exam.

Answers are found at the end of each book, with the correct option screened. Accompanying the correct answer is a discussion of why the other options are incorrect. This allows for even the wrong answers to provide you with a valuable learning experience.

Blackwell has been fortunate to work with expert editors and residents—people like you who have studied for and passed the Boards. They sought to provide you with the very best practice prior to taking the Boards.

We welcome feedback and suggestions you may have about this book or any in the *Blueprints* series. Send to blue@blacksci.com.

All of the authors and staff at Blackwell wish you well on the Boards and in your medical future.

ACKNOWLEDGMENTS

The contributors wish to acknowledge and express their gratitude to Melissa Hardy for her diligence and patience in assisting them in the preparation of this book.

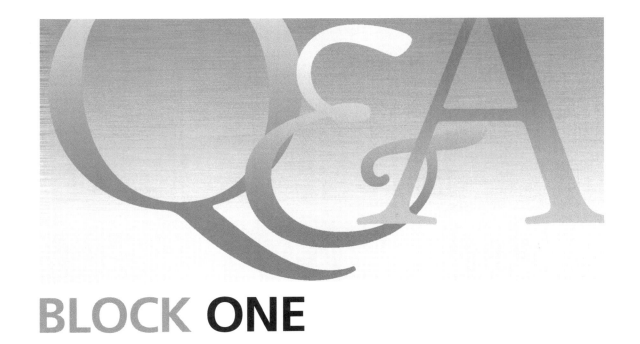

BLOCK ONE

QUESTIONS

QUESTION 1

Regarding the epidemiology of attention deficit hyperactivity disorder (ADHD) all of the following are true EXCEPT:

A. DSM-IV prevalence rates are in the 3–5% range for school age children

B. Male to female sex ratio of 1:3

C. High rate of comorbidity for other psychiatric disorders

D. Risk factors of lower socioeconomic status

E. High incidence of alcoholism as adults

QUESTION 2

Secondary problems associated with attention deficit hyperactivity disorder (ADHD) include which of the following?

A. Social withdrawal and substance abuse

B. Parental abuse

C. Normal adult functioning

D. Accident proneness

E. All of the above

QUESTION 3

Piaget's preoperational thought stage of development includes all of the following EXCEPT:

A. Development of symbolic functions

B. Use of language

C. Deductive reasoning

D. Egocentrism

E. Observational learning

QUESTION 4

For each developmental psychology theorist, select his model of personality formation.

A. Jean Piaget

B. Eric Erikson

C. George Vaillant

D. Sigmund Freud

E. John Bowlby

Attachment theory

Psychosocial tasks

Psychosexual stages

Cognitive stages

Defense mechanisms

QUESTION 5

Each of the following statements about aging and health care is true EXCEPT:

A. Nearly 13% of the current U.S. population are older than 65 years.

B. Very old people constitute one of the fastest growing subgroups within the population.

C. Death rates for heart disease and stroke increased during the past two decades.

D. Only 5% of the elderly reside in nursing homes.

E. 97% of persons age 65 or older are enrolled in Medicare.

QUESTION 6

Each of the following regarding alcohol abuse in the elderly is true EXCEPT:

A. Community prevalence for men is in the 3% range

B. Increased prevalence of mood disorders

C. Respond as well as middle-aged alcoholics to treatment

D. Is differentiated from alcohol dependence by tolerance

E. Commonly has its onset after retirement

QUESTION 7

A 19-year-old female is brought by her mother to the emergency room for dehydration. She appears severely undernourished, and requires intravenous fluids for orthostatic hypotension. She is currently in a treatment program for anorexia. Her laboratory values show a critical hypokalemia. In addition to adding potassium to her fluids, you should:

A. Ask the patient's permission to contact the facility to verify she is in treatment.

B. Recommend that her belongings be searched with her permission for pharmaceuticals.

C. Prescribe thiamine, folate, and a multivitamin daily until nutrition is improved.

D. All of the above.

E. None of the above.

QUESTION 8

A 23-year-old man who is struggling with finishing college is diagnosed with schizophrenia. He eventually drops out of college and loses contact with his family. He is found 5 years later living in a homeless shelter. This illustrates the concept of:

A. Downward drift

B. Dissociation

C. Antisocial behavior

D. Malingering

E. Somatization

QUESTION 9

A 30-year-old male smoker with an 18-pack-year history comes to your office complaining of a dry, hacking cough. You perform a physical examination and obtain a chest X-ray to confirm that he does not have an active infection. You wish to educate the patient about smoking cessation and advise the patient to stop smoking. Which of the following would be the most appropriate first step for intervention?

A. Confront the patient about his smoking behavior and associated health risks.

B. Educate the patient about physiological and psychosocial therapies available for smoking cessation.

C. Establish a therapeutic alliance with the patient.

D. Make a referral to a psychiatrist for nicotine dependence.

E. Give the patient pamphlets on smoking cessation.

QUESTION 10

Dysfunction within the pictured darkened areas of the brain are associated with which psychiatric disturbance?

A. Short-term memory impairment

B. Remote memory impairment

C. Anomia

D. Attention deficits

E. Emotional disturbances

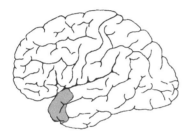
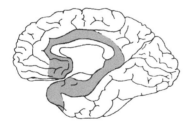

FIGURE 10

QUESTION 11

Psychiatric symptoms associated with multiple sclerosis include each of the following EXCEPT:

A. Depression

B. Mania

C. Compulsions

D. Reduced information processing

E. Memory impairment

QUESTION 12

Fragile X syndrome is associated with each of the following characteristics EXCEPT:

A. More common in females

B. Most common form of inherited mental retardation

C. Involves the long arm of the X chromosome

D. Can be diagnosed with a blood test

E. Treatment is limited to symptomatic management

QUESTION 13

Which of the following statements regarding clinical depression is TRUE?

A. The age of onset has become later in life over the past several decades.

B. The overall rate of depression has decreased in the US.

C. The DSM-IV diagnostic criteria include a six-week duration of the symptoms.

D. A relative lack of dietary W-3 fatty acids has been associated with this condition.

E. This condition is equally common in males and females.

QUESTION 14

A 43-year-old female secretary is followed by her psychiatrist for recurrent annual depressive episodes. She recently watched a special on the local public television channel about seasonal affective disorder (SAD) and is inquiring what causes this condition. The correct response would include each of the following EXCEPT:

A. There are many theories regarding the causes of SAD.

B. Melatonin may be involved.

C. Serotonin may be involved.

D. Diminished appetite seen in winter SAD suggests an endocrine problem.

E. SAD is more common in the northern latitudes.

QUESTION 15

A 34-year-old woman presents to her obstetrician's office accompanied by her spouse three weeks after delivering a healthy infant son. Her husband relates that soon after leaving the hospital his wife has become increasingly irritable, tearful, and is having trouble sleeping. The past week she has become extremely indecisive and expresses concerns that she is not capable of caring for her newborn even though this is her third child. Which of the following is the likely diagnosis?

A. Postpartum blues

B. Puerperal psychosis

C. Postpartum major depression

D. Adjustment disorder with mixed emotional features

E. Bipolar disorder

QUESTION 16

Risk factors associated with the development of postpartum affective disorders include each of the following EXCEPT:

A. History of mood disorder

B. Higher socioeconomic status

C. Complicated pregnancy

D. Thyroid dysfunction

E. Difficult delivery

QUESTION 17

A 30-year-old man presents with the typical findings of depression and is started on an antidepressant medication. At the time of presentation he was having suicidal thoughts, but he had no plan to act on them and felt hopeful about improving with medication. He sees you in your office for a follow-up visit the following week and reports improvement in appetite, sleep, and concentration. He reports having more energy to get up and go to work in the mornings. He still has suicidal thoughts, but they are much less frequent. He still feels he won't act on them. One week later the patient commits suicide. What is the most likely reason that this patient committed suicide after getting treatment?

A. Antidepressant medications can cause some patients to act on suicidal thoughts.

B. The patient is overly stressed by his work and should have been given a work release.

C. Patients are at highest risk for suicide when they begin to regain their energy.

D. Patients frequently feel more hopeless after seeing a psychiatrist and will overdose on the medications they are given.

E. None of the above.

QUESTION 18

A patient that you are starting on valproic acid has a history of elevated ammonia levels in the past when taking this medication. There are no other options at this point in her treatment, so you make the following recommendation:

A. Follow liver function tests every 2 weeks.

B. Place the patient on a stimulant if symptoms return.

C. Start lactulose to prevent an elevated ammonia level this time.

D. Start carnitine to prevent an elevated ammonia level this time.

E. None of the above.

QUESTION 19

A 75-year-old female presents to the emergency room with a broken hip and is given an analgesic for pain relief. Her medications include a monoamine oxidase inhibitor, phenelzine, which she has taken for many years. Shortly after receiving the analgesic she becomes nauseated, diaphoretic, and her blood pressure increases to 190/110. What analgesic was responsible for this reaction?

A. Meperidine

B. Ibuprofen

C. Morphine

D. Codeine

E. Acetaminophen

QUESTION 20

Each of the following is associated with conversion disorder EXCEPT:

A. Extreme concern by the patient for the disability

B. Not intentionally produced

C. Higher incidence in women

D. Frequent history of sexual abuse

E. Symptoms end abruptly

QUESTION 21

An 18-year-old female presents with a fear of having run over someone when she is driving. She has had to stop her car and get out to see if there is a body in the road every time she drives over a bump. When you ask her about other worries, she states she checks her stove, iron, and coffee pot multiple times a day to ensure they are turned off. She has tried to stop doing these things because she feels they don't make sense, but feels intense anxiety if she doesn't stop and check. The medications used to treat this disorder work primarily through which neurotransmitter?

A. GABA

B. Serotonin

C. Glutamate

D. Norepinephrine

E. None of the above

QUESTION 22

A 29-year-old female presents with a 15-year history of drinking. She recently lost her job and is facing DUI charges for the 3rd time in the past 5 years. She asks you to prescribe disulfiram for her because she has met many people in A.A. who have stayed sober after using it. In reviewing the side effects with her you explain that if she ingests any alcohol she may experience flushing, tachycardia, nausea, diaphoresis, or severe anxiety. These symptoms occur because disulfiram causes:

A. An accumulation of acetaldehyde

B. A sudden increase in serotonin levels

C. A decrease in the release of endogenous opioids

D. A sudden decrease in serotonin levels resulting in a panic attack

E. None of the above

QUESTION 23

Alcohol-induced amnestic disorder is associated with each of the following EXCEPT:

A. Also known as Korsakoff's syndrome

B. Related to thiamine deficiency

C. Associated with diffuse brain lesions of the prefrontal cortex

D. Usually picked up with a mental status examination

E. May result in permanent psychosis

QUESTION 24

Each of the following statements about the designer drug Ecstasy is true EXCEPT:

A. Hyperthermia and electrolyte imbalance are side effects.

B. The dosage of the drug is indicative of the outcome.

C. Is closely related to methamphetamine.

D. Is often mixed with heroin and ketamine.

E. Frequent use decreases the experience of euphoria.

QUESTION 25

Each of the following statements about tobacco use is true EXCEPT:

A. 55% of the population experiment with tobacco.

B. The mesolimbic system is involved in the reinforcing effects of nicotine.

C. 30% of smokers succeed in quitting smoking.

D. Smoking is more common among depressed patients.

E. Genetic influences predispose to smoking persistence.

QUESTION 26

Each of the following statements about cannabis usage is true EXCEPT:

A. Regular usage will not lead to dependence.

B. Delirium can occur with long-lasting usage.

C. Cannabis-induced anxiety is a common effect.

D. Decreased libido is associated with regular usage.

E. Delta-9-tetrahydrocannabinol causes the psychoactive effects.

QUESTION 27

Which one of the following neuropsychiatric conditions is best reflected by the sleep stage histogram depicted below?

A. Alzheimer's disease

B. Healthy young adult

C. Parkinson's disease

D. Depression

E. None of the above

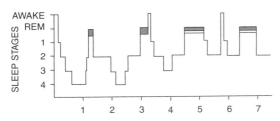

FIGURE 27

QUESTION 28

Which one of the three marked curves best demonstrates the male sexual response with appropriate control?

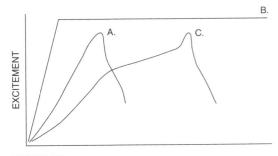

FIGURE 28

QUESTION 29

An IQ in the 40–54 range would be categorized by which one of the following labels?

A. Profound retardation

B. Severe retardation

C. Moderate retardation

D. Mild retardation

E. Borderline retardation

QUESTION 30

A 10-year-old boy is brought to your office by his mother. He has had stomachaches, headaches, and crying spells since school started in the fall. His mother reports this being most severe on Monday mornings while getting ready for school. He feels fine in the afternoons, evenings, and over the weekends, but continues to have physical complaints on school mornings, requesting to stay home from school. He has good friends at school and has never been a discipline problem. After further medical history is obtained and a physical exam is done there is no obvious medical explanation for his symptoms. The most likely diagnosis is:

A. Major depressive disorder

B. Truancy

C. School phobia

D. Antisocial personality disorder

E. Conduct disorder

QUESTION 31

A 7-year-old boy is brought to a psychiatrist because he is doing poorly in first grade. He doesn't seem to pay attention to the teacher, and has not made any friends. He is fascinated with insects and has spent almost all of the last two months in class looking at a book with pictures of insects in it. He had no delay in his language skills and converses normally, but limits his discussions to details about insects. In the office, he makes no eye contact and twirls his hair around his finger. His parents state he has always been like this. What is the likely diagnosis?

A. Asperger's disorder

B. Autistic disorder

C. Obsessive-compulsive disorder

D. Schizophrenia

E. Childhood disintegrative disorder

QUESTION 32

A 9-year-old child is brought for evaluation of his throat. He clears his throat so often that it is disruptive in class and children are beginning to make fun of him at school. His medical evaluation shows no abnormalities. In speaking to him you also notice that he blinks very frequently, but can stop it when asked to. He has already seen a psychiatrist in the past for treatment of his attention deficit and obsessive-compulsive disorders. His mother is concerned and asks what the best treatment for this behavior would be. You make the following diagnosis and treatment recommendation:

A. Conduct disorder—set up a reward system for appropriate behaviors.

B. Tourette's syndrome—begin a medication to lessen episodes while the child is in class.

C. Tardive dyskinesia—stop all psychiatric medications.

D. Generalized anxiety disorder—refer for psychotherapy to decrease overall anxiety level.

E. None of the above.

QUESTION 33

A 15-year-old male is brought in to the Adolescent Clinic by his mother. The mother complains that he had recently been put on suspension from school for frequent fights he initiated with other peers and vandalism of school property. He frequently takes his mother's money from her purse without permission and then denies that he has stolen the money. He has been grounded for staying out past curfew, but sneaks out of the home to see friends. The patient states his mother is "overreacting." The mother feels his behavior has been unmanageable since he was 10 years old.

Which of the following is the most likely diagnosis?

A. Oppositional defiant disorder

B. Autistic disorder

C. Conduct disorder

D. Antisocial personality disorder

E. Attention deficit disorder

QUESTION 34

A 9-year-old girl is brought in by her parents, who state that she has been having terrible nightmares recently. Several nights in the last few months, she has woken up the whole family with her bloodcurdling screams. When this occurs, she seems inconsolable and disoriented, crying and hyperventilating for some time, refusing to acknowledge her parents' presence, and crying until she falls back asleep. The girl admits she is concerned about this, but can't remember what the nightmares were about. On further history, she says that she is generally happy. She admits that her dog dying last year was stressful for her, but denies that it bothers her much now. What is the diagnosis?

A. Post-traumatic stress disorder, with delayed onset

B. Nightmare disorder

C. Panic disorder

D. Sleep terror disorder

E. Temporal lobe epilepsy

QUESTION 35

A 17-year-old male student is uncooperative for his required annual physical. Though he is willing to give adequate history, he is unwilling to disrobe for the physical examination. You notice that he avoids eye contact and appears flushed when you address him for questions. He is wearing four layers of clothing, despite the warm spring weather. Hesitantly, he tells you he hates his "puny" body and does not want anyone to look at it. He says he feels "unmanly" and is on a special diet to "bulk up." He spends hours checking himself and "grooming" in front of the mirror. He admits that he is preoccupied by his body image and he is always comparing his body to other peers. Which of the following would be the most likely diagnosis for this patient?

A. Anorexia nervosa

B. Body dysmorphic disorder

C. Obsessive-compulsive disorder

D. Gender identity disorder

E. Social phobia

QUESTION 36

The negative symptoms of schizophrenia include each of the following EXCEPT:

A. Anhedonia

B. Apathy

C. Asociality

D. Attentional impairment

E. Auditory hallucinations

QUESTION 37

A 60-year-old man has been admitted to the psychiatric unit for psychosis. After visiting one day with his sisters he reports they have been replaced with imposters. He asks to see them through the window before letting them in the unit the next time so that he can determine if they are his "real" sisters or the imposters. This syndrome is called:

A. Folie a deux

B. Amok

C. Capgras

D. Paranoia

E. None of the above

QUESTION 38

Erotomania is a psychiatric syndrome which includes each of the following features EXCEPT:

A. A subtype of the broader DSM-IV classification delusional disorders

B. The attraction to another person is purely sexual

C. Is more common in females in clinical settings

D. Is more common in males in forensic settings

E. May escalate to violence when there is perceived rejection

QUESTION 39

A 48-year-old female nurse was recently admitted for evaluation of recurrent skin infections and sepsis. On review of her medical records, she has been treated for a non-healing abscess on her left forearm as well as her right calf. The medical staff has been particularly suspicious of her recurring infections and noted that she has missed many days of work as a result of needed hospitalizations. Nursing staff later uncovered a syringe that was concealed by the patient in her personal belongings. It was suspected that the patient has been injecting foreign material under the surface of her skin. Which of the following statements is true about a patient with factitious disorder?

A. The symptoms are not intentionally produced by the patient.

B. The patient tends to be overly compliant with medical staff.

C. The motivation for the patient's behavior is to assume the sick role.

D. The motivation for the patient's behavior is to avoid legal responsibility, such as going to work.

E. None of the above.

QUESTION 40

A 28-year-old unemployed white female presents to a psychiatrist for the treatment of anxiety. She states that for the last ten years, she has felt anxious in social situations because other women stare at her. When asked why they stare at her, she states, "I'm not sure, but they might be jealous of my beautiful hair." She denies auditory or visual hallucinations, thought broadcasting, insertion, or withdrawal, but admits that she has "a sixth sense" about people, and that she can sometimes make events happen by thinking about them. She has no friends, though she wishes she did, and in fact has no social contacts other than her mother. As she relates this, she is smiling. She speaks with a British accent, though she states she grew up in Ohio and has never been outside the Midwest. Her speech is organized and coherent, however. What is the likely diagnosis?

A. Schizophrenia, undifferentiated type

B. Paranoid personality disorder

C. Social phobia, generalized type

D. Schizotypal personality disorder

E. Schizoid personality disorder

QUESTION 41

A 32-year-old female singer in a rock group is evaluated for "mood swings." She says that her mood has gone from the "depths of blackness" to "floating on air with happiness" and back several times a day every day for the past twenty years. She also complains of constant anxiety, which is relieved only when she is performing on stage. She denies any history of substance abuse. She has had an extensive number of relationships with men, none lasting more than a few months. She brags about her ability to get men to buy her whatever she wants. On examination, she is wearing heavy make-up and a low-cut shirt, and refers to the doctor as "honey." Her affect is labile, shifting rapidly from tears to laughter and back. What is the most likely diagnosis?

A. Histrionic personality disorder

B. Narcissistic personality disorder

C. Borderline personality disorder

D. Bipolar I disorder

E. Substance abuse

QUESTION 42

Which of the following patients does this chart best represent?

A. Student who presents with abrupt onset of bipolar disorder that partially resolves with treatment

B. Student who presents with abrupt onset of depression that resolves with treatment

C. Student who presents with a "double depression" that partially resolves with treatment

D. Student who presents with a dysthymic episode that resolves with treatment

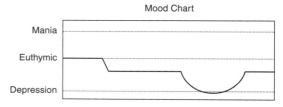

FIGURE 42

QUESTION 43

A 33-year-old male has had a one-month history of depressed mood. He tells you he had an increase in his appetite with an 8-pound weight gain. He is sleeping most of the day. He reports the evening being the most difficult time of day for his mood. His concentration is impaired, and he no longer enjoys watching television or reading like he used to. He feels guilty about how his work has suffered, and is hopeless about being able to recover from this in time to save his job. He denies feeling suicidal, but has had more thoughts of death in the past week. You diagnose him with atypical depression based on which of the following symptoms being present?

A. Increased appetite and sleep

B. Poor concentration and guilt

C. Thoughts of death without suicidal ideation

D. Anhedonia

E. Reversal of diurnal variation in mood

QUESTION 44

A 40-year-old man presents with problems remembering things at work. His children have told him that they find themselves having to repeat information in conversations with him. He has never had memory problems before but has had a stressful year since the death of his father. He is an otherwise very healthy man. He has had loss of appetite, insomnia, and a lot of guilt concerning his father's death from a stroke. What is the most likely cause of this patient's memory problems?

A. Vascular dementia

B. Alzheimer's dementia

C. Encephalopathy

D. Pseudodementia of depression

E. None of the above

QUESTION 45

A 44-year-old female comes to your office for a second opinion. She says she is being treated for bipolar disorder but doesn't understand why she is hearing voices even when she no longer is depressed or manic. On reviewing her records you discover that she has auditory hallucinations and paranoia that never clear completely despite being without any mood symptoms for long periods of time. You inform the patient that your diagnosis would be:

A. Schizoaffective disorder

B. Schizophrenia, residual type

C. Schizophrenia, paranoid type

D. Schizophrenia, disorganized type

E. Major depression with psychotic features

QUESTION 46

A 23-year-old female presents to her employee health services complaining of severe anxiety. She reports symptoms of shortness of breath, sweaty palms, shakiness, and lightheadedness over the past few weeks. She states that she has a work-related presentation scheduled that week as well as an office holiday party that she is expected to attend. She admits that she worries excessively that she will do something to embarrass herself in either of these situations. She has avoided office parties in the past because she thinks others will scrutinize her appearance or behavior. She is distressed because she has few friends and prefers to stay at home rather than go out and meet new people.

A. Social phobia

B. Depression

C. Paranoia

D. Simple phobia

E. Agoraphobia

QUESTION 47

A 19-year-old receptionist presents to her gynecologist with mild symptoms of anxiety and shyness. On physical examination she notices that the patient has only penciled-in eyebrows and no eyelashes. The remainder of the physical examination is normal. The most likely diagnosis is which of the following?

A. Conversion disorder

B. Stereotypical movement disorder

C. Schizophrenia

D. Factitious disorder

E. Trichotillomania

QUESTION 48

A 28-year-old woman presents to a psychiatrist for evaluation of "bad thoughts." She relates that for the past three years, she has been plagued by thoughts of harming her husband. Every day, many times throughout the day, she experiences detailed visual images of stabbing him repeatedly with a kitchen knife, or of him lying bloody and mangled as she runs him over with her car. She is very upset about and ashamed of these images, as she states that she loves her husband, does not want to hurt him, and would never act on these images. She attempts to ignore or suppress them, but they are completely beyond her control. She identifies them as her own thoughts, however. She denies auditory hallucinations, thought insertion, broadcasting, or withdrawal, delusions of control, or other paranoid phenomena. She denies any repetitive behaviors or mental acts which she feels driven to perform and she denies a history of violent behavior. On examination, she appears extremely distressed and anxious but her thought process is organized and logical. What is the most likely diagnosis?

A. Schizophrenia, undifferentiated type

B. Sexual sadism

C. Partner relational problem

D. Dissociative disorder, not otherwise specified

E. Obsessive-compulsive disorder

QUESTION 49

A 26-year-old single woman is referred by her primary care physician to a psychologist for testing. An MMPI is performed resulting in a "conversion V" profile as reported on the 1, 2, and 3 scales. Which one of the following conditions is most closely associated with this profile on the MMPI?

A. Psychosis

B. Somatoform disorder

C. Invalid profile

D. Normal profile

E. None of the above

QUESTION 50

A 47-year-old man has presented to his primary care doctor eight times in the last year with concerns over a variety of minor symptoms such as dry skin, vague abdominal discomfort, and so on. He states he was in good health prior to the age of 46. At each visit, full history, examination, and appropriate lab testing reveal no physical abnormality. His doctor repeatedly reassures him of this. When the doctor does this the patient believes him, but before long he again becomes concerned about a new symptom. The symptoms themselves are less troubling to him than is the fear he feels that he might have some serious, unknown medical illness which the doctor has missed finding. On questioning, he has no other psychiatric symptoms. Though this concern about having an unknown illness is obviously genuine and very distressing to him, he never requests time off work, hospitalization, or inquires about medical disability payments. What is the likely diagnosis?

A. Delusional disorder, somatic type

B. Somatization disorder

C. Hypochondriasis

D. Malingering

E. Major depressive disorder

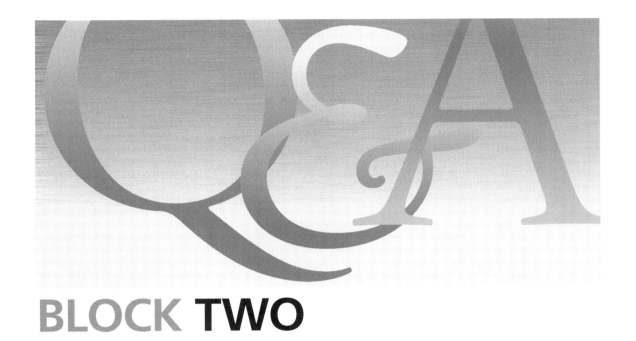

BLOCK TWO

QUESTIONS

QUESTION 51

Each of the following statements about anorexia nervosa is true EXCEPT:

A. Anorexia nervosa is present in all cultures.

B. The rate of this illness is higher in women than men.

C. Amenorrhea may precede significant weight loss.

D. Depression is a frequent comorbid illness.

E. Lack of insight is frequent.

QUESTION 52

A 30-year-old female patient, who visits the urgent care clinic frequently, complains of a "burning sensation" during sexual intercourse. She has no pregnancy history and has a normal physical and pelvic exam. Her medical record indicates that she has been in for multiple physical complaints with no evidence of disease by repeated examinations. In order to make the diagnosis of somatization disorder, her complaints over the past several years should consist of the following EXCEPT:

A. At least one sexual or reproductive symptom

B. Complaints related to a medical condition that are in excess of what would be expected from history, exam, and laboratory findings

C. History of depression or anxiety

D. Significant impairment in social, occupational, or other significant areas of functioning

E. At least one neurological symptom

QUESTION 53

A 68-year-old man is asked to reproduce the face of a clock correctly, demonstrating the hours from 1 to 12. Which one of the following neuropsychiatric disorders is most consistent with his drawing?

A. Subcortical dementia and parkinsonism

B. Schizophrenia

C. Attention deficit disorder

D. Pseudodementia of depression

E. Multiple sclerosis

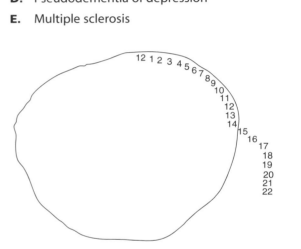

FIGURE 53

QUESTION 54

A 59-year-old female presents to the emergency room after coming to work very confused. She had difficulty answering questions, and her coworkers saw her stumbling. Her coworkers are puzzled because she doesn't seem to smell of any alcohol. They report repeated episodes of the patient coming to work intoxicated and state she has been alcoholic for most of her life. On exam you find her disoriented with a disconjugate gaze and staggering gait. The diagnosis that is most consistent with this presentation and most worrisome is:

A. Acute alcohol intoxication

B. Transient ischemic attack

C. Wernicke's encephalopathy

D. Korsakoff's syndrome

QUESTION 55

A 23-year-old male student presents with a six-month history of extreme daytime fatigue and repeatedly falling asleep in classes, on the bus, and other inappropriate places. On review of systems, he admits to sometimes "fainting" when he is upset. He describes these fainting spells as a sudden feeling of weakness, causing him to fall down, but with preserved consciousness throughout. On further questioning which of the following symptoms are also likely to be present in this patient?

A. Somnambulism (sleepwalking)

B. Hallucination-like dreams

C. Cogwheel rigidity

D. Loud snoring

E. Palpitations

QUESTION 56

Which of the following EEG patterns best reflects REM sleep?

A.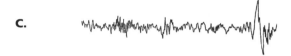

B.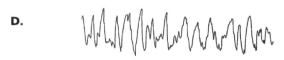

C.

D.

E.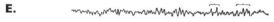

FIGURE 56

QUESTION 57

Which of the following is true of the biopsychosocial model of approaching illness?

A. It emphasizes the structural and chemical nature of disease.

B. It emphasizes the cognitive, psychodynamic, and personality factors affecting disease.

C. It emphasizes the role of one's culture, support system, and living environment on disease.

D. All of the above.

E. None of the above.

QUESTION 58

A 74-year-old male comes to your office for a routine checkup. He has been a patient of yours for many years and has never been a management problem. Near the end of the visit he tells you he is very angry at his neighbor. He has been able to hear all of his neighbor's thoughts for the past week and believes the man has been monitoring him with hidden cameras. He further informs you that he has bought a shotgun and intends to shoot the man the next time he comes out to complain about his yard. When you ask him if he is serious about this he replies, "You bet I am." After a prolonged discussion about this and repeated efforts to resolve the problem otherwise, he tells you, "I don't care what happens to me legally, I'm going to shoot him in the leg and teach him a lesson." You are obligated to:

A. Respect the patient's confidentiality and do nothing.

B. Try to talk him out of it, and document that clearly in the chart before you let him leave the office.

C. Obtain an outpatient evaluation of the patient by a psychiatrist later that week.

D. Arrange an emergency evaluation.

E. None of the above.

QUESTION 59

A 12-year-old boy is brought into the office by his mother for symptoms of anxiety and checking behaviors. His mother gives a normal birth history and states that the boy's developmental milestones were normal from birth. From age 4, she notes that he has been easily distracted and extremely overactive for his age. At age 7 he was given the diagnosis of ADHD and was treated with methylphenidate. His anxiety was noted only recently and appears to be associated with the need for symmetry and counting rituals. On evaluation, the boy displayed motor tics of excessive blinking, head turning, and repetitive foot stomping. He would frequently clear his throat and repeatedly grunt or sniff. When these behaviors were brought to the attention of the mother, she stated, "Oh yes, he does that all the time, but so does his father." Which of the following medications would be most helpful to treat the patient's motor and vocal tics?

A. Haloperidol

B. Clonazepam

C. Fluoxetine

D. Dextroamphetamine

E. Clomipramine

QUESTION 60

A 23-year-old patient presents to your office with complaints of depression. He has trouble sleeping, poor appetite, feelings of hopelessness, and passive suicidal ideation with no plan. He recently lost his job because he has been chronically late or missing many days of work. The patient reports that he would be late because he would need to check the parking brake on his car several times, as well as return to his car several times to make sure it was locked. He was embarrassed to admit that he missed work on days that he knew his coworkers had cold symptoms. He was fearful that he would catch their germs and become violently ill as a result. You also notice that the patient's hands are dry and irritated. The patient explains that he washes his hands frequently throughout the course of the day to avoid contamination.

Which of the following would be the best form of medication treatment for the patient?

A. Bupropion

B. Desipramine

C. Nefazodone

D. Fluvoxamine

E. Nortriptyline

QUESTION 61

Which one of the graphed curves best reflects the relationship between clinical response and the plasma levels for nortriptyline?

A. Curvilinear

B. Sigmoidal

C. Straight line

D. None of the above

E. All of the above

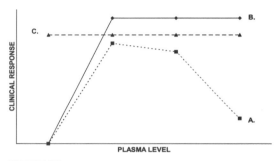

FIGURE 61

QUESTION 62

Which one of the graphed curves best reflects the relationship between clinical response and the plasma levels for imipramine?

A. Straight line

B. Sigmoidal

C. Curvilinear

D. None of the above

E. All of the above

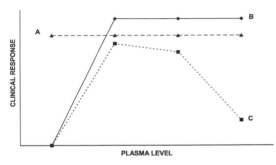

FIGURE 62

QUESTION 63

A 30-year-old man is admitted to a locked psychiatric unit for court-ordered treatment, after threatening to kill himself. He gives a three-week history of irritable mood, sleep fragmentation, high energy, loss of appetite, a ten pound loss of weight, and racing thoughts. He states that he has had six episodes like this in the past year. He has a five-year history of bipolar disorder and is currently taking valproic acid and paroxetine. On examination, he is restless, his speech is pressured, and his affect is labile. Which of the following would NOT be an appropriate intervention at this time?

A. Urine drug screen

B. Stopping the paroxetine

C. Stopping the valproic acid

D. Electroconvulsive therapy

E. Milieu therapy

QUESTION 64

A 36-year-old male presents to your office with rapid speech, elevated mood, increased energy, poor sleep, and increased appetite. You consult a psychiatrist who recommends initiating medication treatment with lithium. The psychiatrist asks you to perform some baseline tests before starting the medication. All of the following tests should be done to appropriately monitor the patient taking lithium EXCEPT:

A. Baseline EKG

B. CBC

C. Liver enzyme panel

D. TSH

E. BUN and creatinine level

QUESTION 65

A 30-year-old female presents to your office for follow-up on her obsessive-compulsive disorder and depression. She has decided to try to get pregnant and wants to know if she has to stop taking her fluoxetine. She had a severe suicide attempt 1 year ago and has had severe peripartum depression in the past. You recommend:

A. Continue the fluoxetine since the risks of harm to the baby from the medication are small.

B. Continue the fluoxetine despite the risks of heart or neural tube defects since her history is so concerning.

C. Stop the fluoxetine and watch for a recurrence of symptoms.

D. Stop the fluoxetine and if depression occurs she will have to receive electroconvulsive treatments.

E. None of the above.

QUESTION 66

A 23-year-old unemployed female who is four months pregnant is brought to an emergency room by police after they had found her standing on a bridge over a freeway threatening to jump. She tells the doctor that for the last six weeks she has felt severely anxious and depressed, waking in the early hours of the morning. She has not eaten or drunk for four days because she is extremely worried that demons have poisoned her food and water. She admits to frequent use of IV heroin and cocaine until four weeks ago. She is dehydrated and disheveled, wearing soiled clothing and displays considerable psychomotor retardation. Which of the following is the MOST appropriate treatment option to initiate at this time?

A. Clonazepam, 0.5 mg tid

B. Electroconvulsive therapy

C. Carbamazepine, 200 mg bid

D. Intensive cognitive-behavioral therapy

E. Intensive chemical-dependency treatment

QUESTION 67

A 30-year-old female presents to your office after being evaluated in the Emergency Room for chest pain. She reports that her medical workup for heart disease was negative, but that she continues to have episodes of chest pain and fears she is going to have a heart attack. On further evaluation, you identify her episodes as lasting usually 10 minutes and associated with shortness of breath, sweating, lightheadedness, tingling in her extremities, and an intense feeling of doom. After educating the patient about the symptoms of panic disorder, you suggest medication treatment. All of the following medications may be helpful in treating her symptoms EXCEPT:

A. Bupropion

B. Alprazolam

C. Sertraline

D. Imipramine

E. Phenelzine

QUESTION 68

A 43-year-old female presents to the Emergency Room with severe anxiety. She reports that she had been taking alprazolam up to four times a day for panic attacks. Over the past few days, her anxiety symptoms are worse and she complains of trouble falling asleep and nausea. On further evaluation, she admits that she had recently skipped her regular doses because a friend told her that the medication she is taking is addicting. Which of the following would be the most appropriate intervention:

A. Discontinue alprazolam and switch her treatment with a serotonin reuptake inhibitor.

B. Refer patient back to her outpatient physician.

C. Switch the patient to a longer-acting benzodiazepine, such as clonazepam.

D. Educate patient on proper use of her medication, risks and signs of benzodiazepine withdrawal.

QUESTION 69

A 30-year-old woman presents with depression. She has had no prior episodes, but did see a psychiatrist one year ago because of bulimia. She states she still occasionally purges. You decide that she does need antidepressant treatment and discuss many options with her. The one medication that you would hesitate to recommend in this patient would be:

A. Buspirone

B. Nefazodone

C. Sertraline

D. Bupropion

E. Fluoxetine

QUESTION 70

A 45-year-old man is evaluated for insomnia and anxiety. He dates the onset of his symptoms to one year ago, when he received a concussion in a car accident while working. In spite of a normal MRI scan of his brain taken on the day of the accident, he has suffered from headaches, dizziness, difficulty concentrating, poor memory, fatigue, insomnia, anxiety, and depressed mood. Once asleep, he frequently awakens with nightmares about the accident. He feels "jumpy," and is short-tempered with his wife and coworkers. Driving, especially, is an ordeal for him, making him feel tense and irritable. He has missed six months of work in the past year because of these symptoms.

Which of the following diagnoses would be the LEAST likely?

A. Post-traumatic stress disorder

B. Post-concussional disorder

C. Malingering

D. Acute stress disorder

E. Chronic subdural hematoma

QUESTION 71

A 42-year-old man is admitted to a psychiatric ward and gives a six-month history of severely depressed mood, loss of appetite and weight, insomnia, and auditory hallucinations commanding him to hang himself. While on the ward, he spends his time joking and socializing with other patients, smoking heavily, eating double portions, and sleeping soundly without hypnotic medication. Despite this, he continues to complain of hallucinations and a severely depressed mood, and states he will kill himself if discharged. It is noted that he is homeless, that the weather has been unseasonably cold recently, and that he admits he does not care to live in homeless shelters, citing how dangerous they can be. What would be the most appropriate option for management of this patient?

A. Start an MAOI, because he has an atypical depression as evidenced by his reactive and apparently normal affect.

B. Order MMPI testing.

C. Restrict smoking privileges until he leaves voluntarily.

D. Have him arrested for fraud.

E. Supply him with a one-way bus ticket to a warmer state.

QUESTION 72

Each of the following patients comes to your office asking if they can stop their medications. Which patient would you feel most comfortable tapering off the medication mentioned?

A. A man with bipolar disorder who is taking valproic acid and has had no episodes for the past year

B. A woman with major depression with psychotic features who has had no psychotic symptoms for the past 3 months on haloperidol and intends to stay on her antidepressant

C. A man with schizoaffective disorder treated with olanzapine who has had no psychotic symptoms for the past 3 months

D. A schizophrenic man on risperidone who has just gotten a job after 3 years of minimal psychotic symptoms

QUESTION 73

An 88-year-old woman is seen by her primary physician for difficult to control hypertension and prior cerebral vascular accidents. Her current blood pressure reading is 160/95 mmHG. She has continued to be depressed since her last stroke despite an adequate trial of paroxetine. The physician asks you if the antidepressant he is planning to switch her to is safe with her medical history. Which medication may need to be avoided if possible in this patient?

A. Nefazodone

B. Venlafaxine

C. Fluoxetine

D. Sertraline

E. Bupropion

QUESTION 74

Which of the following types of psychotherapy is most efficacious for treating panic disorder?

A. Psychodynamic psychotherapy

B. Cognitive-behavioral therapy

C. Interpersonal psychotherapy

D. Psychoanalytic psychotherapy

E. None of the above

QUESTION 75

The focus of dialectical behavioral therapy (DBT) for patients with a borderline personality disorder includes each of the following EXCEPT:

A. Accepting the patients the way they are while trying to teach them to change

B. Encompassing cognitive and behavioral therapy approaches

C. Identifying alternative responses to stressful events

D. Uncovering unconscious conflicts

E. Skills training in the areas of interpersonal effectiveness and emotional regulation

QUESTION 76

A psychiatrist is consulted to see a 29-year-old woman who is being treated in an ICU for complications resulting from her intentionally overdosing on her medication. This is her fourteenth overdose in the past five years. All of them have been desperate attempts to stop various boyfriends from leaving her. Several of the ICU nurses complain that she is being mistreated by other nurses. They accuse these nurses of labeling her a "problem patient" despite her "sweet and vulnerable nature," and of punishing her by ignoring many of her requests for care, and otherwise being rude to her. The accused nurses admit that she is indeed a difficult patient, but that despite her constant verbal abuse and hostility toward them, they have at all times been very polite to her. What would be the most appropriate management of the situation?

A. Report to the head of nursing that the ICU nursing team is unprofessional and unable to work together.

B. Tell the patient that next time she overdoses, she will have to go to another hospital.

C. Call a meeting for the nurses, and invite a professional conflict mediator to help resolve their dispute.

D. Call a meeting for the nurses, and explain the concept of splitting.

E. Establish a token economy for the patient as a behavioral treatment.

QUESTION 77

The principles of sleep hygiene management include each of the following EXCEPT:

A. Take a nap during the day

B. Exercise early

C. Wake up at your usual time

D. Go to bed at your usual time

E. Abstain from stimulants

QUESTION 78

For each constellation of symptoms, select the most likely diagnosis.

A. Major depressive disorder

B. Delirium

C. Schizophrenia

D. Delusional disorder

E. Bipolar disorder

F. Panic disorder

G. Obsessive-compulsive disorder

H. Generalized anxiety disorder

I. Anorexia

J. Bulimia

QUESTION 78A

A 23-year-old underweight woman with amenorrhea, osteoporosis, lanugo, bradycardia, infantile uterus, and cold intolerance.

QUESTION 78B

A 63-year-old man two days post-operative for prostate surgery abruptly experiences disorientation, visual hallucinations, tachycardia, fever, and motor restlessness.

QUESTION 78C

A 32-year-old single mother experiences recurrent episodes of trembling, chest discomfort, dizziness, chills, and paresthesias.

QUESTION 78D

A 53-year-old successful defense lawyer complains of symptoms of fatigue, poor appetite, lessened sleep, and decreased libido. He is contemplating retiring, expressing concern that his poor performance in court has let several clients down.

QUESTION 78E

A 20-year-old single man is reluctantly brought to the office by his parents, with whom he has lived all his life. He has no complaints. His parents relate for the past several years their son has essentially remained at home with no regular social contacts or activities. He occupies himself reading science fiction comic books. Occasionally he will blurt out the phrase "It doesn't matter" but will not explain to whom he is speaking or responding.

QUESTION 78F

A 36-year-old grade school teacher is referred by her gynecologist for treatment of depression. In developing her personal history she acknowledges at least three two-week episodes of decreased need for sleep, hypersexuality, and buying sprees. There is no history of substance abuse.

QUESTION 78G

A mildly overweight 24-year-old secretary requests diuretics to relieve her abdominal bloating. Further information gathering reveals a history of severe weight fluctuations since age 14. She now eats excessively two or three times a week but has learned to compensate by using laxatives and diuretics.

QUESTION 78H

A 23-year-old receptionist presents to her family physician very distressed that she is about to be fired. In asking her why, she relates arriving at work later and later each day because she must return home to make sure her curling iron has been turned off and the doors of her house locked.

QUESTION 78I

A 63-year-old divorced woman presents to the emergency center very distressed that her neighbor of 5 years is spying on her through a telescope. Her concerns began only a month ago. Her mental status examination is otherwise normal and she denies any substance abuse.

QUESTION 78J

A 56-year-old developer relates to his new primary care physician a lifelong history of being fretful and nervous with frequent bouts of insomnia when he is more worrisome. There is no particular focus to his anxieties. He relates years of psychoanalysis as well as biofeedback and relaxation training have been unhelpful.

QUESTION 79

Each of the following personality disorders is followed by correct descriptions of expected associated behaviors EXCEPT:

A. Paranoid: wariness, suspicion, jealousy, and violence

B. Schizoid: submissive, clinging, and indecisive

C. Antisocial: deceiving, manipulative, and seeking secondary gains

D. Borderline: impulsive, angry, and poor sense of reality

E. Narcissistic: entitled, vicious, and competitive

QUESTION 80

For each grouping of physiologic side effects, select the most likely medication class.

A. Dry mouth, sedation, tachycardia, tremor, and weight gain

B. Sexual dysfunction, nausea, diarrhea, and headache

C. Galactorrhea, amenorrhea, akathisia, and weight gain

D. Sedation, ataxia, weakness, and anterograde amnesia

E. Thirst, tremor, diarrhea, and goiter

QUESTION 80A

Lithium

QUESTION 80B

Tricyclic antidepressants

QUESTION 80C

Selective serotonin reuptake inhibitors (SSRIs)

QUESTION 80D

Benzodiazepines

QUESTION 80E

Antipsychotics

QUESTION 81

A 23-year-old single male with the diagnosis of chronic undifferentiated schizophrenia is brought to the emergency center by the paramedics with hyperthermia, severe muscle rigidity, autonomic instability, and delirium.

Which class of psychiatric medications has this patient most likely been recently exposed to, causing these clinical symptoms?

A. Benzodiazepines

B. Tricyclic antidepressants

C. Selective serotonin reuptake inhibitors

D. Monoamine oxidase inhibitors

E. Antipsychotics

QUESTION 82

Which of the following is NOT considered a potential treatment for NMS?

A. Dantrolene

B. Discontinue all antipsychotic medications

C. Bromocriptine

D. Amantadine

E. Valproic acid

QUESTION 83

A 43-year-old chronically mentally ill man was admitted to the medical floor for ketoacidosis. His previously prescribed antipsychotic haloperidol was stopped and not restarted when he was transferred to an extended care facility several weeks later. A routine follow-up examination by his primary care physician finds the patient with tic-like movements of his face and tongue and lip smacking. Based on this information, what is the most likely diagnosis?

A. Diabetic neuropathy

B. Tourette's disorder

C. Parkinson's disease

D. Akathisia

E. Tardive dyskinesia

QUESTION 84

Which one of the following predisposing factors for tardive dyskinesia (TD) is INCORRECT?

A. Advanced age

B. Male gender

C. Mood disorders

D. Family history of affective disorders

E. Exposure to several antipsychotic medications

QUESTION 85

Which of the following have not been beneficial in treating tardive dyskinesia?

A. Clozapine

B. Vitamin E

C. Propranolol

D. Haloperidol

E. Tetrabenazine

QUESTION 86

A 26-year-old law student is referred to a psychiatrist by her family physician for treatment of symptoms of severe anxiety, frequent hand-washing, and hoarding. She relates to the consulting psychiatrist that she has experienced a variety of obsessions and compulsions since age 10.

Which of the following statements about obsessive-compulsive disorder (OCD) is INCORRECT?

A. Concordance between monozygotic twins is negligible.

B. The condition affects between 2% and 3% of the population.

C. Presents at a younger age in males than females.

D. Symptoms most commonly include cleaning, arranging, counting, and checking.

E. Patients are often secretive regarding the nature and extent of their obsessions and compulsions.

QUESTION 87

OCD is distinguished from other anxiety disorders by the presence of which of the following symptoms?

A. Phobias

B. Compulsions

C. Obsessions

D. Exaggerated startle response

E. None of the above

QUESTION 88

After validating the referring physician's diagnosis of OCD for this patient, the consulting psychiatrist recommends a specific pharmacologic treatment. Which is the best class of psychotropic medications to choose from?

A. Anticonvulsants

B. Benzodiazepines

C. Selective serotonin reuptake inhibitors

D. Antipsychotics

E. Beta blockers

QUESTION 89

Which of the following is NOT a common side effect seen with SSRIs?

A. Delayed ejaculation

B. Headache

C. Nausea

D. Extrapyramidal symptoms

E. Anorgasmia

QUESTION 90

Considering the patient's long history of OCD symptoms, the consulting psychiatrist also recommends psychotherapy for her. Which of the following choices is likely to be most helpful?

A. Cognitive-behavioral therapy

B. Psychodynamic psychotherapy

C. Group therapy

D. Interpersonal psychotherapy

E. Existential therapy

QUESTION 91

For each group correlate the percentile incidence of schizophrenia.

A. 47%

B. 8%

C. 1%

D. 39%

E. 12%

91A. Both parents schizophrenic

91B. General population

91C. Sibling schizophrenic

91D. One parent schizophrenic

91E. Monozygotic twin schizophrenic

QUESTION 92

A 63-year-old retired teacher shared with his primary care physician (PCP) during a routine office visit that he has noticed increasing difficulty with his memory. Otherwise he is in good health and requiring no medication.

Which one of the following psychological tests is a valuable screening device to be used by primary care physicians in this type of situation?

A. MMPI

B. WAIS

C. Thematic Apperception Test

D. Mini-Mental State Exam

E. Rorshach Tests

QUESTION 93

While performing the Mini-Mental State Exam the PCP asks her patient to copy the following design. What cognitive function is being assessed by this request?

A. Language

B. Orientation

C. Registration

D. Recall

E. Visual-motor integrity

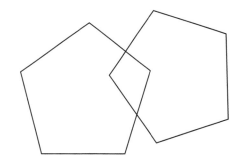

FIGURE 93

QUESTION 94

A 23-year-old, otherwise healthy, single woman presents to the emergency center complaining of an episode of lightheadedness, chest discomfort, shortness of breath, and trembling, which occurred earlier that morning and lasted nearly 10 minutes. This is the first episode of these symptoms, but she is very fearful that it will happen again.

Each of the following psychiatric conditions are commonly associated with her symptoms EXCEPT:

A. Agoraphobia

B. Depression

C. Avoidant personality

D. Substance abuse

E. Mania

QUESTION 95

Upon further questioning the patient relates she had three cups of strong coffee just before the onset of symptoms.

Of the following, which agent is associated with producing panic symptoms?

A. Isoproterenol

B. Serotonin

C. Lactic acid

D. Inhalation of carbon dioxide

E. All of the above

QUESTION 96

Which of the following treatment interventions would be LEAST likely to alleviate panic symptoms?

A. Decrease her caffeine intake

B. Paroxetine

C. Amitryptyline

D. Haloperidol

E. Alprazolam

QUESTION 97

Each of the following statements about alcohol withdrawal is true EXCEPT:

A. The withdrawal syndrome occurs once the blood alcohol level reaches zero.

B. Symptoms typically last 2–7 days.

C. Repeated periods of withdrawal may exacerbate the severity of future episodes of withdrawal.

D. The severity of symptoms depends on the amount and duration of alcohol consumption.

E. Seizures can occur in major as well as minor withdrawal states.

QUESTION 98

After being started on thiamine, folate, and multivitamins, the patient is admitted to the inpatient unit. Laboratory studies are normal except for several abnormal liver function tests.

Which of the following class of medications is indicated for this type of alcohol-withdrawing patient to prevent further withdrawal symptoms?

A. Anticonvulsants

B. Beta blockers

C. Antipsychotics

D. Long-acting benzodiazepines

E. Short-acting benzodiazepines

QUESTION 99

Seventy-two hours after being admitted the patient develops delirium tremens.

Which one of the following statements about delirium tremens is NOT true?

A. Typical symptoms include gross tremor, confusion, fever, hallucinations, and incontinence.

B. Auditory hallucinations are more common than visual hallucinations.

C. Occurs in 5% of patients admitted for withdrawal.

D. Has a 15% mortality rate.

E. Typically occurs 3–5 days after the patient stops drinking.

QUESTION 100

Select the BEST CHOICE of the expected neuropsychiatric deficits and symptoms resulting from head trauma to each of the identified areas of the brain:

A. Loss of memory and nominal dysphasia

B. Disorders of body image and ideational deficits

C. Disinhibition and apathy

D. Color agnosia

E. None of the above

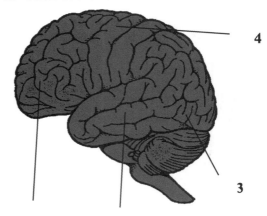

FIGURE 100

QUESTION 100A

Region 1

QUESTION 100B

Region 2

QUESTION 100C

Region 3

QUESTION 100D

Region 4

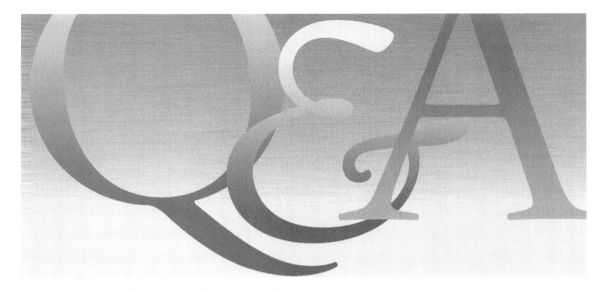

BLOCK ONE

ANSWERS

ANSWER 1

B. ADHD is far more common in boys than girls, with a sex ratio of approximately 3:1. Although prevalence rates can be affected by changing the threshold number and severity of symptoms, most experts agree on the 3–5% range. Comorbid psychiatric conditions may include conduct, oppositional, and anxiety disorders. Half of Tourette's patients have comorbid ADHD which usually precedes the tics. Many with ADHD later develop alcohol and drug problems.

ANSWER 2

E. All of the above. In addition to the primary symptoms of inattention, hyperactivity, and impulsivity, ADHD can cause secondary problems. Poor attention to social cues can cause a child to be unpopular and rejected by peers. Parental frustration in repeatedly disciplining the child can result in abuse. Hyperactivity combined with impulsiveness and inattention to danger and warnings makes children with ADHD accident-prone. The adult outcome of ADHD is variable. At least one-third are not significantly different in adulthood from a matched normal control group. Another 20–30% develop alcohol or drug problems in adulthood.

ANSWER 3

C. Deductive reasoning is developed during the later adolescent years during the formal operations stage. Preoperational development typically occurs in the pre-school years and also includes thinking by intuition and differentiation between signs and symbols.

ANSWER 4

Attachment theory

E. John Bowlby. A British psychoanalyst, Bowlby's work focuses on animal ethology and evolutionary theory.

Psychosocial tasks

B. Eric Erikson. A German-born psychoanalyst, Erikson expanded Sigmund Freud's psychosexual theories to include social and cultural dimensions.

Psychosexual stages

D. Sigmund Freud. Considered the founder of modern psychiatry, Freud described the oral, anal, and genital phases as fundamental to psychological development.

Cognitive stages

A. Jean Piaget. A Swiss child psychologist, Piaget theorized cognitive and intellectual functioning as central to personality development.

Defense mechanisms

C. George Vaillant. Vaillant's work categorized ego mechanisms of defense as primitive, immature, neurotic, and mature from infancy through adulthood.

ANSWER 5

C. The death rates for heart disease and cerebrovascular disease have been declining while the rates of death due to cancer have increased. By the year 2030 one in three Americans will be 55 years or older. The "very old," classified as those older than 85 years, are one of the fastest growing groups. Among persons reaching age 60 by 1990, more than one-half of the women and one-third of the men are expected to enter a nursing home eventually. Not surprisingly, the absolute number and percentage of the population benefiting from Medicare continues to rise.

ANSWER 6

E. Although 30% of people with alcoholism older than age 65 began their abuse after age 60, the majority established their pathological use earlier. The 3% prevalence rate typically includes institutionalized elderly patients. Alcoholism is associated with higher prevalence of both mood and cognitive disturbances. Tolerance is seen with continuous alcohol use, leading to a dependence on increased consumption. The principles of treatment for elderly alcoholics are similar to younger patients. Late-onset drinkers have a better response rate to treatment.

ANSWER 7

D. Due to the lethality of this case an effort should be made to ensure appropriate treatment is actively being pursued. Since many patients with an eating disorder will abuse laxatives or diuretics that lower their potassium to critical levels, the facility should be informed, if the patient permits, to look for contraband. This patient is high risk for nutritionally based diseases and should be supplemented.

ANSWER 8

A. The downward drift hypothesis is based on the belief that persons with mental illness tend to drift into a lower socioeconomic class because their illness interferes with skills needed to maintain a higher socioeconomic status. There is a slow drift downward as living skills become more and more impaired.

ANSWER 9

C. Establishing a therapeutic relationship is important due to the chronic, relapsing nature of nicotine dependence. Advising a patient to stop smoking is best done in a supportive and non-judgmental manner. There are currently no studies to support that confrontational styles are effective for smoking cessation. Often smokers are ambivalent about quitting, and giving more personalized information and feedback on smoking cessation can increase motivation to change.

ANSWER 10

E. The darkened areas represent the cortical components of the limbic system. The common feature shared by limbic system dysfunction is an emotional disturbance. Psychosis, mood disorders, obsessive-compulsive behavior, personality alterations, and disturbances of sexual behavior are linked to limbic system dysfunction.

ANSWER 11

C. Compulsions are *not* particularly associated with MS. Depression is the most common psychiatric symptom associated with this population, with a lifetime prevalence of 40–50%. Suicide risk is also elevated. The coexistence of mania and MS is as high as 13 times what would be expected in a normal population. Steroid therapy may precipitate manic episodes, but there is evidence that underlying organic changes in the brain play a role. Cognitive deficits such as memory impairment, slowed information processing, and concentration problems become present in 60–70% of MS patients.

ANSWER 12

A. Fragile X syndrome is more common in males than females, affecting 1 in 2000 and 1 in 4000, respectively. It is the most common inherited form of mental retardation and second only to Down's syndrome as a cause of mental impairment. As the name implies, the syndrome is the result of a fragile site on the long arm of the X chromosome attributed to the excess amplification of the trinucleotide CGG sequence. It is thought that the protein produced by this gene is responsible for guiding the connections between neurons involved in learning and memory. The symptoms of this pervasive developmental disorder include mental retardation ranging from learning disabilities to severe intellectual impairment, hyperactivity, unstable mood, and autistic-like behaviors. The diagnosis can now be made by a DNA probe to pinpoint the defective gene. Presently gene repair is not possible, so treatments include behavioral and pharmacologic management of the symptoms.

ANSWER 13

D. Over the past century, the sharp increase in the dietary intake of W-6 (omega) fatty acids and a rapid decline of dietary W-3 (omega) fatty acids has paralleled the increased rate of depression in the US. Interestingly there has been a progressive earlier age of onset, as well, while the condition remains more prevalent in women compared to men. DSM-IV diagnostic criteria include a depressed mood or decreased interest for at least two weeks with the associated symptoms of sleep and appetite changes, energy disturbance, guilt, poor concentration, and suicidal ideation. Clinical depression is thought to affect 11 million Americans yearly.

ANSWER 14

D. Diminished appetite is not typical of SAD. In fact, carbohydrate craving is common for winter SAD. The theories regarding SAD are numerous, emanating from observation, clinical research, and patient intuition. The incidence of pure SAD is much higher in the northern latitudes, resulting in an interest in the seasonal variations of sunlight exposure and temperature as possible causes. The administration of melatonin can cause relapses in patients with SAD. The most accepted theory as to the etiology of SAD involves serotonin. The more common successful treatments for SAD affect serotonin in some way. These include the selective serotonin reuptake inhibitors (SSRIs) and light therapy.

ANSWER 15

C. Postpartum major depression. The postpartum period is a time of increased risk for development of mood disturbances in women. Postpartum depressive disorders are divided into three classifications: postpartum blues, postpartum depression, and puerperal psychosis. Postpartum blues is the most common and is separated from postpartum depression by the severity of symptoms in the latter condition and typically peaking within the first week after delivery. Postpartum or puerperal psychosis is relatively rare, with the onset for the majority of cases within 2 weeks postpartum. Psychotic symptoms would include delusions, hallucinations, and bizarre, disorganized behavior. There is an association between postpartum psychosis and bipolar disorder. This patient's symptoms are too severe to classify as an adjustment disorder. Her mood disturbance warrants psychiatric consultation and likely will require pharmacologic treatment.

ANSWER 16

B. Higher socioeconomic status. Actually, a lower socioeconomic status with antecedent chronic stress, inadequate social supports, limited funds for basic needs such as food, formula, shelter, etc. is a risk factor for postpartum mood disorders. Women with a history of postpartum affective disturbances have a recurrence rate as high as 50% in some studies. For this population, medical and psychologic prevention prior to delivery is very important. In some cases, prophylactic antidepressants or mood stabilizing agents are warranted. Thyroid dysfunction itself can cause a mood disorder, and certainly a complicated delivery can be traumatic psychologically.

ANSWER 17

C. In a severe depression there is characteristically a loss of drive, concentration, and energy to carry out any plans. As these factors improve, it becomes possible that the patient will develop and carry out a plan for suicide.

A. This is a misperception because of the effect that they have on improving the patients' vegetative symptoms.

B. That is not necessarily so, since some patients do better if they are distracted and still involved in their normal activities.

D. Patients frequently report more hope after seeing a psychiatrist, which is part of the placebo response seen in antidepressant medications and therapy.

ANSWER 18

D. The mechanism that leads to elevated ammonia levels in patients taking valproic acid is based on a depletion of the vitamin carnitine which is required in fatty acid transport. If carnitine is depleted by valproic acid, it can disrupt this process, which results in ammonia formation. Some patients can prevent this from occurring by taking carnitine as a supplement. Unfortunately it does not reverse the process for everyone. Of note, the degree of ammonia elevation is not an accurate indicator of expected severity of symptoms.

A. The liver function tests are not indicators of this specific problem.

B. This is not the treatment for high ammonia levels.

C. Lactulose decreases ammonia levels in alcoholics by increasing transit time in the bowel, which reduces the amount of ammonia that is transported across the bowel wall to the serum. This is minimally helpful in patients with valproic acid induced elevations in ammonia.

ANSWER 19

A. Meperidine (Demerol) is contraindicated in patients taking monoamine oxidase inhibitors. It can result in a serotonin syndrome that can include severe hypertensive crisis, occipital headache, stiff neck, sweating, nausea, restlessness, muscle twitches, seizures, and high fever. Morphine and codeine in high doses or in a patient on other potentiating medications could lead to this syndrome as well, but meperidine is the most likely culprit.

ANSWER 20

A. Many conversion disorder patients exhibit *la belle indifference*, a lack of concern regarding an apparent extreme decline in their health. This condition often presents in late adolescence or early adulthood and is more common in women with histrionic personality disorder and past history of sexual abuse during childhood. In contrast to malingering or factitious disorder, the symptoms of a conversion disorder are not intentionally produced, but rather the ego defense mechanisms of repression and dissociation are unconsciously at work. The symptoms generally begin suddenly following a period of psychological stress and in most cases end abruptly and are of a short duration.

ANSWER 21

B. Obsessive-compulsive disorder is thought to occur due to serotonin dysregulation. The areas of the brain that are thought to be involved are the frontal lobes, the basal ganglia, and the cingulum. Treatment includes selective serotonin reuptake inhibitors such as fluvoxamine or fluoxetine, or the tricyclic agent clomipramine.

ANSWER 22

A. The fear of the unpleasant symptoms of disulfiram is used as a deterrent to future drinking in those patients who are willing to take the medication. It works by causing a shift in the chemical reaction involved in metabolizing alcohol in the liver. The result is a shift toward the production of acetaldehyde. Severe reactions can occur if a patient drinks despite taking her disulfiram. In those cases an alternative method must be used.

B. The toxic effects of disulfiram are not a result of serotonin level changes.

C. An alternative agent to disulfiram is naltrexone, an opiate antagonist, which works by decreasing cravings and rates of relapse.

D. Though the sensation after ingesting alcohol is described like a panic attack, the mechanism of action of disulfiram is not thought to be through serotonin pathways.

ANSWER 23

C. At autopsy, patients with Korsakoff's syndrome show hemorrhage and sclerosis of the mammillary bodies and thalamic nuclei along with diffuse lesions of the brain stem, cerebellum, and limbic system. Thiamine treatment is usually successful in treating this condition, which can be diagnosed clinically by the presence of cognitive deficits and confabulation. One-fourth of patients with this condition remain impaired chronically.

ANSWER 24

B. The dosage of Ecastsy (3,4 methylenedioxy-methamphetamine or MMDA) is not always indicative of the outcome. Small amounts have resulted in hyperthermia and near death. This drug can cause a serotonin-like syndrome requiring rapid cooling of the body. The associated dancing in a warm environment at a "rave party" can result in severe electrolyte imbalance as well. Frequent users may develop tolerance to the pleasant or euphoric effects of MMDA. Other drugs may be added to produce or augment the psychotropic effect being sought.

ANSWER 25

C. Only 2–3% of dependent smokers succeed in quitting smoking. Tobacco use for many is a classical addictive disorder with the behavior pattern of compulsive drug use despite adverse psychosocial and health consequences. Dopamine is the key neurotransmitter of the mesolimbic system reinforced by nicotine stimulation. Some research suggests that the effects of nicotine may have similar results as antidepressants. This may explain the shared benefit of the antidepressant bupropion for smoking cessation. Both genetic and environmental factors are important to develop regular tobacco use. Those who persist smoking have a .70 genetic predisposition.

ANSWER 26

A. Cannabis or marijuana used regularly can lead to dependence and withdrawal. Persistent use despite psychological and physical impairment as well as developing tolerance are hallmarks of such. The delirium seen with cannabis is similar to what is seen with the hallucinogens and psychomimetics and can last up to 10 days. Decreased libido, ataxia, increased reaction time, perceptual distortion, and restlessness are also associated with cannabis usage. Anxiety is common during acute intoxication, especially for inexperienced users, and is often provoked by paranoid thoughts. Although there are approximately 60 active substances in cannabis, THC is thought to be the key chemical responsible for the psychoactive effect.

ANSWER 27

B. The depicted histogram is that typically seen in a healthy young adult. REM sleep (darkened area) occurs cyclically through the night, and stages 3 and 4 (slow wave sleep) are concentrated earlier during sleep. Alzheimer's disease is typically marked by frequent interruptions in sleep throughout the night. Parkinson's disease is plagued by an increased number of awakenings throughout the night, as well, with decreased REM sleep. Sleep disturbances are seen in most patients with major depression and are characterized by sleep fragmentation and a redistribution of REM sleep into the first half of the night.

ANSWER 28

C. In comparison to curve A and curve B, curve C demonstrates greater voluntary control over ejaculatory reflex. Although graph B may initially be construed as desirable in that there is no identified ejaculation, retarded or delayed ejaculation can be painful and distressing. Various medications can produce an inability to ejaculate, including psychotropics such as serotonin reuptake inhibitors.

ANSWER 29

C. Moderate retardation is the correct answer. The IQ is a standardized score of the Wechsler Adult Intelligence Scale (WAIS) with a population mean of 100 and a standard deviation of 15. A score less than 25 is labeled profound retardation; 25–39, severe retardation; 55–70, mild retardation; and 70–80, borderline retardation. The WAIS is designed for people 16 years and older. The Wechsler Intelligence Scale for Children and a Wechsler Preschool and Primary Scale of Intelligence are used for younger individuals.

ANSWER 30

C. School phobia is characterized by symptoms being most severe in the mornings while getting ready for school. Typically the child's somatic symptoms and feelings of distress are most severe after a long weekend away from school, and they tend to reduce as the child progresses through their day at school. It is necessary to determine if there is a justified fear such as the child being bullied or teased. If no medical or situational explanation is found, it is important to keep the child attending school as much as possible. If the child faces the anxiety consistently, it will likely extinguish and the school phobia will resolve.

A. Depression may lead to a school avoidance over time, but other symptoms of depression should be present throughout the day and on weekends.

B. Truant children will readily leave the home claiming they are going to school.

D. Antisocial personality disorder cannot be diagnosed before the age of 18 and is characterized by a disregard for and a violation of others' rights.

E. Conduct disorder is the appropriate term for antisocial characteristics before the age of 18; however, the history doesn't support a discipline problem.

ANSWER 31

A. Patients with Asperger's disorder have impaired social interaction and restrictive, repetitive behaviors and interests but normal language skills.

B. The features of autistic disorder are similar to Asperger's disorder, but also include impaired language skills. Asperger's disorder is thus considered to be a less severe variant of autism.

C. In OCD, repetitive behaviors and interests may also be present, but these are intended to prevent or reduce distress in some way. Social skills are not primarily affected.

D. This patient does not demonstrate psychotic features such as delusions, hallucinations, or disorganized thought processes, which are required for the diagnosis of schizophrenia.

E. Childhood disintegrative disorder is a syndrome of loss of previously acquired skills in language, behavior, bowel or bladder control, play, or motor skills.

ANSWER 32

B. The classic triad in children is Tourette's syndrome, obsessive-compulsive disorder, and attention deficit disorder. These three disorders are seen so frequently together that if one is found during an evaluation, the other two disorders should be screened for as well.

A. No evidence that this is conduct related.

C. No antipsychotic medications are mentioned, nor are they routinely used in the treatment of this child's other psychiatric disorders.

D. No symptoms of generalized anxiety disorder are mentioned.

ANSWER 33

C. There is a persistent pattern of behavior that violates the basic rights of others or societal norms or rules. Behaviors include either aggression toward others, destruction of property, deceitfulness or theft, and serious violations of rules, beginning in childhood.

A. ODD consists of a pattern of negativistic, hostile, and defiant behaviors. Opposition toward authority figures is demonstrated by persistent disobedience, argumentativeness and violation of minor rules. Legal violations are more characteristic of conduct disorder.

B. In autistic disorder, aggressive behavior does not necessarily lead to a violation of the basic rights of others.

D. Antisocial personality disorder develops in adolescence but is diagnosed when the individual is 18 years or older.

E. Although attention deficit disorder may be seen in such an individual, impulsive behavior does not necessarily lead to a violation of rules or the basic rights of others.

ANSWER 34

D. Sleep terror disorder is characterized by episodes of awakening from sleep with a scream, accompanied by intense fear and autonomic arousal, with unresponsiveness to others during the episode, and subsequent amnesia for the episode.

A. In PTSD, the traumatic event remains a focus of the person's symptoms; for example, with persistent intrusive recollections of the event, avoidance of reminders of it, and persistent symptoms of increased arousal.

B. In nightmare disorder, the patient rapidly becomes oriented and responsive on wakening, and remembers the nightmares.

C. Panic attacks may wake patients from sleep, but there is rarely a history of screaming or disorientation.

E. Fear is sometimes a feature of the aura of temporal lobe seizures, and post-ictal confusion is the rule, but most such seizures start with motionless staring, followed by lip smacking. Screaming and crying during a seizure would be quite unusual.

ANSWER 35

B. Dysmorphic disorder is characterized by preoccupation with an imagined defect or excessive concern of appearance. Preoccupation is marked by distress or impairment in social functioning.

A. Though the patient is preoccupied with the size of his body, the preoccupation is not limited to fear of "fatness." The patient is on a special diet in order to "bulk up" or gain weight.

C. Though rituals are commonly seen in BDD, the rituals are limited to preoccupation with the imagined defect.

D. Preoccupation with primary or secondary sexual defects is characteristic of gender identity disorder. However, this individual appears to desire being "more manly" in his appearance and does not express desire to be more like the opposite sex.

E. In both disorders there is fear of rejection and humiliation; however, it is clear that this patient's fear of humiliation is limited to his imagined body defect.

ANSWER 36

E. Auditory hallucinations are considered positive symptoms of schizophrenia, along with ideas of reference, thought broadcasting, and delusional thinking. Although successful treatment of positive symptoms will keep patients out of the hospital, the negative symptoms can be a tremendous handicap to the patients, their families, and society. Converse to the hyperdopaminergic hypothesis of positive symptoms, negative symptoms may involve hypodopaminergic activity in the frontal lobes of the brain.

ANSWER 37

C. Capgras' syndrome describes a specific delusion that is seen mostly in schizophrenic patients. The patient believes that a person has been replaced with an exact double that can act in every way like the original. It is named after the psychiatrist who first described the delusion.

A. This describes a delusion that begins in one patient and becomes incorporated into a significant other's beliefs and behaviors so that they eventually share the delusion.

B. This is a Malayan term for a sudden fury and violent behavior developing in a person.

D. This is a broad term for this type of delusion. The more specific answer is Capgras' syndrome.

ANSWER 38

B. The central theme of erotomania is a delusional belief that another person is in love with them in an idealized, romantic way rather than a pure sexual attraction. Most mental health experts believe erotomania is underdiagnosed because people with this condition do not seek psychiatric treatment. Stalking behavior can occur in erotomania. Violence is more common in males with erotomania and occurs more frequently when there are multiple objects of the delusional fixation and a history of antisocial behavior. The erotomaniac stalks to gain the idealized relationship and can react violently when the delusional beliefs are threatened.

ANSWER 39

C. Factitious disorder is characterized by intentional production or feigning of physical or psychological symptoms of a medical condition. Motivation for the behavior is to assume the sick role.

A. Symptoms that are not intentionally produced by a patient to assume the sick role would be more characteristic of a somatoform disorder.

B. A patient with factitious disorder is more often demanding and disruptive with medical staff. These individuals will often dispute lab results and sign out against medical advice when confronted with a negative medical workup.

D. External incentives such as avoiding legal obligations, responsibilities, or just seeking a room for the night are absent in factitious disorder. Malingering would be the proper term for this behavior.

ANSWER 40

D. Individuals with schizotypal personality disorder appear eccentric, with their odd ideas, magical thinking, inappropriate affect, and persistent social anxiety. They are usually socially isolated, but may gravitate toward fringe groups or subcultures, where their personality style may appear less unusual.

A. Schizophrenia by DSM-IV definition must include two or more symptoms of delusions, hallucinations, disorganized speech or behavior, and negative symptoms (affective flattening, avolition, etc.). The patient is uncertain of her belief that other women might be jealous of her hair, and therefore this does not qualify as a delusion.

B. Patients with paranoid personality disorder are suspicious of others without basis, but

do not have the odd ideas, magical thinking, and other eccentricities of schizotypal patients.

C. In social phobia, anxiety is associated with negative evaluations of the self, rather than with the paranoid fears about others typically seen with schizotypal personality disorder.

E. Unlike this patient, schizoid patients do not desire to have friends.

ANSWER 41

A. The attention-seeking behavior of patients with histrionic personality disorder manifests in a number of ways: through exaggerated displays of emotion, use of dramatic expressions in speech, use of their physical appearance to draw attention to themselves, and inappropriate familiarity and seductiveness. Because they are uncomfortable in situations where they are not the center of attention, they sometimes gravitate toward the entertainment industry.

B. Patients with narcissistic personality disorder share histrionic patients' need for admiration, but their presentation is dominated by a grandiose sense of self-importance.

C. Borderline personality disorder is also notable for affective instability and dramatic, unstable relationships, but identity disturbance is a key feature and the characteristic affect displayed is one of inappropriate anger.

D. Many psychiatrists would consider this patient to have a bipolar spectrum illness because of her mood lability. However, the bipolar I diagnosis rests on the presence of a history of a full-blown manic episode, a seven-day period of elevated or irritable mood, along with symptoms of neurovegetative disturbance.

E. Substance abuse is possible despite her denial. However, the history overall is characteristic for histrionic personality disorder, so that remains the most likely diagnosis.

ANSWER 42

C. A double depression is a major depressive episode that occurs in the setting of dysthymia. For prognostic reasons it is important to determine if dysthymia co-exists since dysthymia may result in a longer treatment time or higher doses of medication being required.

A. With no hypomanic or manic episodes evident on this chart, one cannot diagnose a bipolar disorder.

B. There is an abrupt depression here, but it only partially resolves to the level of the dysthymia. It is possible for this patient to return to a euthymic mood and have a complete resolution of symptoms; however, this is not seen in this chart.

D. A dysthymia is present both before and after the depressive episode, but only the major depression showed a resolution with treatment.

ANSWER 43

E. Other findings would be mood reactivity to positive events, leaden paralysis, and a pattern of interpersonal rejection sensitivity. Increased appetite and sleep don't distinguish atypical depression, though they are often present. In typical depression the patients describe feeling the worst in the morning and better as the day progresses, which is termed diurnal variation. This patient shows a reversal of that pattern. Diagnosing atypical features can be helpful because it is one of the few indications to specifically choose a monoamine oxidase inhibitor. All of the other answers are findings in "typical" depression.

ANSWER 44

D. This patient, who has no known medical problems and is exhibiting symptoms of depression, is likely having memory problems as a result of a mood disorder. If concentration is impaired by a mood disorder, the patient will have difficulty getting new information into his or her short-term memory. This results in information not making it into long-term memory. Treatment of his mood should resolve his memory problems.

A. Though his father had a stroke, this is an unlikely cause due to his age and the absence of other physical findings.

B. This is a diagnosis of exclusion that requires a mood component to be ruled out, as well as other possible causes of a dementia.

C. No medical conditions are present to support this.

ANSWER 45

A. A bipolar patient has psychosis only during a depression or mania. If psychotic symptoms are present despite full treatment of mood symptoms, the diagnosis is schizoaffective disorder. This impacts your treatment because the patient may need indefinite antipsychotic treatment.

B. This is the term for a chronic schizophrenic who has predominantly negative symptoms such as disorganization, flattened affect, or vegetative symptoms.

C. This is the term for the schizophrenic with the typical spectrum of hallucinations and delusions.

D. This is the term for the schizophrenic who has very disorganized speech, is difficult to understand, and has inappropriate emotional responses.

E. If psychotic symptoms are present when the patient is not depressed, this cannot be the diagnosis.

ANSWER 46

A. Social phobia is an anxiety disorder of persistent fear that one or more social situations will result in humiliation of the individual or scrutiny by others. Affected individuals avoid social or performance situations in fear they will embarrass themselves or be judged as anxious or stupid. Individuals with social anxiety usually experience physical symptoms of anxiety and marked anticipatory anxiety far in advance of upcoming social situations.

B. Social withdrawal is common with depression but is usually associated with a lack of interest rather than fear of social situations.

C. Paranoia is marked by fear that someone will do something untoward to the individual, not that they will be humiliated.

D. Simple phobia is marked and persistent fear of a clearly discernible, circumscribed object or situation, and exposure leads to immediate anxiety response, for example, social situations related to crowds or being in an enclosed space.

E. Agoraphobia is characterized by avoidance of situations due to fear the individual will have incapacitating panic-like symptoms or fear of losing control.

ANSWER 47

E. Trichotillomania is the irresistible urge to pull out one's hair. There is some gratification or relief upon pulling out the hair, but the disturbance causes distress or impairment socially. Onset of this condition usually occurs in the teenage years and is four times more common in females. Some mental health experts consider trichotillomania a variant of obsessive-compulsive disorder, and it is not uncommon to uncover other ritualistic behaviors or obsessions. The clinical course is varied and since the hair pulling may result in chewing or swallowing hair, trichobezoars may be present in the GI tract, resulting in abdominal complaints, iron deficiency anemia, and hair in the stools.

ANSWER 48

E. Obsessions are defined as recurrent intrusive thoughts, impulses, or images that are recognized as inappropriate and are distressing to the patient. This woman is one of the approximately 10% of patients with obsessive-compulsive disorder who have only obsessions, without compulsions.

A. The images are experienced as being her own thoughts, and so do not qualify as hallucinations.

B. In sexual sadism, fantasies of injuring or humiliating others evoke sexual excitement, which is not present in this case.

C. This DSM-IV diagnosis is used when the clinical focus is a maladaptive pattern of interaction between spouses. This does not appear to be the case here.

D. In dissociative disorders, there is a loss of a unitary sense of self or identity. There is no evidence for dissociation here.

ANSWER 49

B. Conversion "V" is a profile seen on the MMPI when there are elevations of hypochondriasis (1) and conversion hysteria (3) scales both higher than the elevated depression (2) scale, resulting in a "V" configuration. This suggests that the patient is depressed but unable or unwilling to interpret the experience psychologically. Distress is typically experienced physically, resulting in nonspecific somatic preoccupations.

ANSWER 50

C. Hypochondriasis is characterized by a preoccupation with fears that one has a serious disease due to an unrealistic assessment of one's symptoms. This fear persists despite reassurance, and is distressing to the patient.

A. In hypochondriasis, the fear of having a serious disease is not of delusional intensity, as seen in patients with delusional disorder, somatic type, who cannot be convinced even briefly that their beliefs are inaccurate.

B. Somatization disorder is characterized by a variety of unexplained symptoms occurring over many years and by definition must begin before age 30.

D. Malingering is the intentional simulation of symptoms and/or signs of illness in order to gain some external incentive, like insurance benefits or time off work.

E. Major depressive disorder by definition includes symptoms of depressed mood or loss of interest or pleasure in life, along with a variety of other symptoms such as sleep disturbance, loss of appetite, and so on.

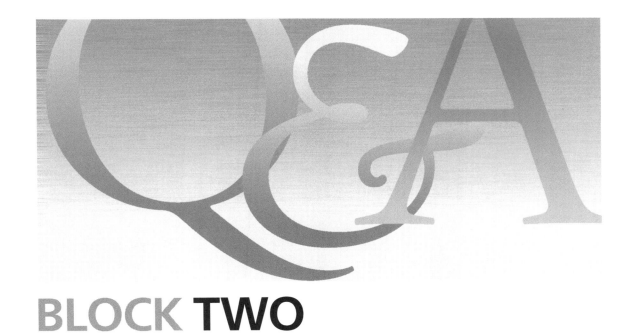

BLOCK TWO

ANSWERS

ANSWER 51

A. Interestingly, anorexia nervosa occurs primarily in industrialized societies where the incidence of starvation is almost nonexistent. The illness is much more common in women, especially in social and vocational environments demanding thinness, such as dancing, modeling, and athletics. Typically reluctant or secretive about their illness, the presence of amenorrhea may be a suspicious clue for the primary care physician to pursue other associated symptoms and behaviors. Obsessive-compulsive traits and depression are common comorbid conditions. It is not unusual for family or friends to bring the anorectic for evaluation due to family concerns rather than the patient's concern.

ANSWER 52

C. Individuals with somatization disorder may experience symptoms of depression or anxiety; however, these symptoms are not always present and are not necessary for the diagnosis. Other criteria needed for the diagnosis of somatization disorder include a history of at least two gastrointestinal symptoms other than pain and four pain symptoms related to four different anatomical sites or functions. Symptoms cannot be explained by a known medical condition or effects of a chemical substance, and symptoms are not intentionally produced or feigned.

ANSWER 53

A. Poor planning and perseveration with micrographia are most consistent with a subcortical dementing process and parkinsonism.

ANSWER 54

C. Wernicke's encephalopathy is characterized by acute confusion, sixth nerve palsy, and unsteady gait. Though the triad is characteristic, it may occur with very subtle eye or gait findings that are initially missed. Since this is potentially reversible it is important to be actively looking for these findings to ensure the diagnosis is not missed.

A. Though it can appear as if the patient is intoxicated, remember that most intoxicated people are not disoriented, nor do they have opthalmoplegia on exam.

B. Patients with thiamine deficiency may have cardiovascular disease, but this would not be a typical TIA presentation. The more worrisome diagnosis is Wernicke's, which can be treated if recognized quickly.

D. Korsakoff's syndrome is a persistent form of thiamine deficiency. It presents more slowly and is characterized as a failure in short-term memory. The patient may confabulate her history to conceal her memory deficits. If Wernicke's encephalopathy progresses to Korsakoff's syndrome, the chances of recovery diminish to only 20%.

ANSWER 55

B. Hallucination-like dreams occurring at sleep onset (hypnogogic hallucinations) or on waking (hypnopompic hallucinations) are often associated with narcolepsy. The most common presentation of narcolepsy is of excessive daytime fatigue and irresistable attacks of refreshing sleep. Cataplexy is also common, and is defined as the sudden loss of muscle tone, usually precipitated by intense emotions.

A. This is a separate sleep disorder.

C. Cogwheel rigidity occurs in parkinsonism.

D. Loud snoring is characteristic of obstructive sleep apnea, which also presents with excessive sleepiness, but is not associated with cataplexy.

E. Palpitations might be associated with syncope, which by definition involves loss of consciousness.

ANSWER 56

E. REM sleep is low voltage with a random, fast pattern including sawtooth waves, marked by brackets on this illustration. Pattern A is an awake state with a random, fast pattern and low voltage as well but without the sawtooth waves. Pattern B shows typical alpha waves seen in a drowsy state. Pattern C has the sleep spindle and K complex patterns seen in Stage 2 sleep. Pattern D illustrates this frequent, exaggerated delta wave seen in delta sleep.

ANSWER 57

D. The biopsychosocial model is an attempt to approach all patients in a comprehensive manner. Reviews of their past medical history, family medical history, physical symptoms, the physical exam, and any laboratory or pathology findings are included in the biologic assessment. Reviews of coping skills, current motivations and goals, and personality traits that may affect the intensity or ability to adapt to the illness are included in the psychological assessment. The person's family and community influences are included in the social assessment. Combined, these factors offer a better sense of how to understand and subsequently treat the problem that the patient is bringing to the physician.

ANSWER 58

D. According to the Tarasoff decision you must report threats of violence where the patient has shown intent toward a specific person or persons. Every reasonable effort should be made to keep the patient in the office until the appropriate safe disposition is made. One should not put oneself in danger, however, to achieve this.

A. Reasons to break confidentiality include homicidal ideation, suicidal ideation, and report or evidence of child abuse.

B. You still have an obligation to protect public safety.

C. The patient could act on his plan by the time the consultation occurs, even if that was the very next day.

ANSWER 59

A. Tourette's syndrome is characterized by chronic motor and vocal tics that begin in childhood. Comorbid psychiatric disorders that are often seen with Tourette's syndrome include obsessive-compulsive disorder (OCD) and attention deficit disorder. Tourette's disorder is up to nine times more common in male children than female children, and family studies suggest that tic disorders share a common genetic etiology. Dopamine antagonists, typically given in low doses, such as haloperidol or pimozide, have been most effective in treating the tics of Tourette's syndrome.

B. Although clonazepam may cause improvement of tics in some patients with Tourette's disorder, it is not the most effective form of treatment.

C. Fluoxetine may be helpful for comorbid symptoms of OCD, but is not known to be helpful for treatment of tics.

D. Stimulants, such as methylphenidate and dextroamphetamine, may actually worsen the tics seen in Tourette's syndrome.

E. Like other serotonin agents, clomipramine has not been shown effective in treatment of tics but may be helpful for comorbid symptoms of OCD.

ANSWER 60

D. The patient exhibits symptoms of obsessive-compulsive disorder and would benefit from treatment with an antidepressant with serotonergic properties. Fluvoxamine is a selective serotonin reuptake inhibitor that has been FDA approved for treatment of OCD.

A. Bupropion is an antidepressant with dopaminergic and noradrenergic properties and has not been shown to be effective in treatment of OCD.

B. Desipramine is a tricyclic antidepressant with highly noradrenergic properties. Clomipramine is an alternative tricyclic antidepressant with serotonergic properties shown to be effective for OCD.

C. Nefazodone antagonizes the 5-HT2 receptor but shows modest blockade of 5-HT reuptake. Studies are lacking that show its effectiveness for treatment of OCD.

E. Nortriptyline is another noradrenergic tricyclic antidepressant.

ANSWER 61

A. There is a curvilinear relationship between clinical response and nortriptyline plasma levels. The clinical response increases with the plasma level but plateaus in the 50–150 ng/ml range. This range is called the therapeutic window. The decreased clinical response above 150 ng/ml is not due to side effects.

ANSWER 62

B. A sigmoidal relationship exists between response and imipramine plus its therapeutic metabolite desipramine levels. This clinical response increases with a plasma level up to approximately 250 ng/ml and then levels off. The antidepressant nortriptyline is associated with a curvilinear clinical response–plasma level relationship.

ANSWER 63

C. The patient is currently having an episode of mania, for which the treatment of choice is a mood stabilizer, such as valproic acid. Stopping it would likely worsen his condition. A blood level should be measured and the dosage optimized. His bipolar disorder is also a rapid cycling one, defined as four or more episodes of a mood disturbance in the past year.

A. Despite his known history of bipolar disorder, abuse of illicit drugs may be playing a role in his current presentation.

B. Antidepressants can initiate mania and they can initiate or worsen rapid cycling. In manic patients and in most patients with rapid cycling, they should be discontinued.

D. Studies suggest that ECT may be more effective than medication for the treatment of mania.

E. Milieu therapy is an important part of inpatient psychiatric treatment and refers to the use of the hospital environment itself as a therapeutic intervention. It includes such techniques as behavioral reinforcement, peer support, and structured scheduling of daily activities.

ANSWER 64

C. Liver enzymes should be monitored in individuals who are taking valproic acid or carbamazepine, but not lithium, which is excreted primarily through the kidney.

A. Lithium may cause EKG changes such as flattening or inversion of T waves or, more seriously, sinus node dysfunction.

B. Elevation of white blood count is possible while taking lithium.

D. Hypothyroidism secondary to lithium can be detected by elevation of TSH.

E. Renal function should be monitored every 3 months initially, then about every 6 months thereafter or when disease is suspected.

ANSWER 65

A. Fluoxetine is second only to the tricyclic agents in studies of antidepressants in the setting of pregnancy. There are no known teratogenic effects with its use throughout the pregnancy or in breastfeeding despite its being present in the breast milk.

B. Lithium is associated with Ebstein's anomaly in the heart, and the anticonvulsants are associated with neural tube defects. These patients must be taken off their medications if found to be pregnant unless symptom severity is severe. Certainly they should be counseled about continuing on these medications if they are trying to get pregnant.

C. Her history is concerning and predicts another episode of peripartum depression is likely, and often the episodes will become more severe with successive pregnancies. Unless she has objections to being on the medication, she should be maintained on her current dose.

D. Electroconvulsive treatments are generally safe in pregnancy, but they are not the only treatment option she has available to her.

ANSWER 66

B. Electroconvulsive therapy (ECT) is considered by many clinicians to be the treatment of choice for severely depressed pregnant women, especially if they are putting themselves and their fetus at high risk by refusing oral intake. ECT is also considered to be particularly effective for psychotic depression, for patients who are acutely suicidal, and for patients with marked psychomotor agitation or retardation.

A. This would be likely to worsen the patient's psychomotor retardation. It would also interfere with ECT, because of its anticonvulsant activity.

C. This is inappropriate for the same reason as clonazepam. Additionally, both carbamazepine and clonazepam are known teratogens.

D. & E. A patient this ill is not likely to be able to participate in these therapies. They would be useful as part of her continuing care, however.

ANSWER 67

A. Bupropion has not been shown to be effective in treatment of panic disorder and does not appear to have antipanic properties. Tricyclic antidepressants, particularly imipramine, and benzodiazepines such as alprazolam have been shown to be effective in treating panic disorder. Selective serotonin reuptake inhibitors, such as sertraline, have valuable antipanic properties and are useful to treat panic disorders. MAOIs such as phenelzine are also very effective in treatment of panic disorder.

ANSWER 68

D. Discontinuation of benzodiazepines, such as alprazolam, can lead to relapse or rebound symptoms of anxiety, or more severe withdrawal symptoms. Rebound symptoms such as anxiety, insomnia, and GI symptoms are milder and short-lived. However, symptoms of withdrawal are more serious, such as agitation, tachycardia, palpitations, blurred vision, muscle cramps, and seizures. In an emergency setting, educating the patient about risks associated with discontinuation of benzodiazepines would be most appropriate and prevent more serious effects.

ANSWER 69

D. The most serious potential side effect of bupropion is seizures. The risk of having a seizure is increased when there is an eating disorder such as bulimia or anorexia. The mechanism is not understood at this time, but if possible an alternative agent should be used in this patient. The other options listed do not have a contraindication with a history of eating disorders.

ANSWER 70

D. Acute stress disorder is similar to post-traumatic stress disorder, but by DSM-IV definition, lasts a maximum of 4 weeks.

A. & B. With this history, the patient meets criteria for both post-traumatic stress disorder and post-concussional disorder as proposed by DSM-IV. The latter diagnosis is recognized by most neurologists and is believed to be attributable to diffuse microscopic shearing injuries to axons, which show up better on post-mortem dissection specimens than they do on MRI.

C. Unfortunately, more so than with most injuries, one must consider malingering when assessing work-related injuries.

E. Subdural hematomata may take weeks to accumulate after head injuries, and thus may not show up on brain imaging done at the time of the accident.

ANSWER 71

B. The Minnesota Multiphasic Personality Inventory assesses a wide range of personality variables, and also rates responses on a "lie scale," an "infrequency scale," and a "suppressor scale," which can be useful in identifying malingering. It would not make a final determination of the patient's degree of truthfulness, but would provide supporting evidence.

A. Patients taking MAOIs must be reliable in following certain dietary restrictions. Since there is some question as to this patient's reliability, an MAOI would be inadvisable.

C., D., & E. These would be risky and questionable ethically. Nicotine withdrawal particularly is extremely uncomfortable—even genuinely ill patients may leave the hospital if smoking is denied them.

ANSWER 72

B. This is a case where you should actively be working with the patient to eventually stop the antipsychotic. The psychotic symptoms should resolve once the condition is adequately treated with an antidepressant. Usually the patient can be tapered off the haloperidol fairly quickly while continuing on the antidepressant. The risk of tardive dyskinesia is reduced by using the antipsychotic for as short a time period as possible, and using an atypical antipsychotic whenever possible.

A. Most bipolar patients will require indefinite treatment with a mood stabilizer to prevent future episodes. If this is not done, it is believed that a "kindling phenomenon" occurs. This refers to the observation that future episodes will occur with progressively less time between them, more severe symptoms, and less of a response to treatment.

C. This patient is at higher risk for a recurrence of symptoms since stabilization of mood is not sufficient to prevent psychosis.

D. His treatment may be more necessary if his stress level is about to increase.

ANSWER 73

B. The most concerning side effect of venlafaxine is a possible sustained elevation of blood pressure. The diastolic may increase to >90 mmHG, and the systolic may increase by 10 mmHG or more from baseline. If this patient's hypertension was well controlled, venlafaxine could be an appropriate choice. The other antidepressants listed do not have this effect.

ANSWER 74

B. Cognitive-behavioral therapy (CBT) can be very helpful in treating panic disorders. Some studies found an equal efficacy to pharmacologic interventions. CBT is based on the premise that panic is a learned response. Cognitive misinterpretations of environmental and internal cues result in a conditioned response, which can be unlearned. Insight-oriented therapies based on underlying unconscious conflicts or unresolved relationship issues tend not to alleviate the specific symptoms of a panic disorder.

ANSWER 75

D. Uncovering unconscious conflicts is a component of psychoanalytic or psychodynamic psychotherapy. DBT is a more practical type of therapy developed by Marsha Linehan and her colleagues aimed at reducing inappropriate behaviors and teaching skills to handle surges of emotion. Strategies include teaching the patient to do a chain analysis of what led up to an identified problematic event and identifying what alternatives could have been taken to avoid the event. Both individual and classroom group scenarios are utilized in DBT.

ANSWER 76

D. Splitting, a primitive defense mechanism where external objects are divided into categories of "all good" or "all bad," is characteristically employed by patients with borderline personality disorder. When hospital staff are unwittingly coopted into these patients' defensive strategies, they may become divided against each other. The ICU nurses should be advised regarding the psychological dynamics of the patient, and on how to manage the countertransference (i.e., the feelings toward her) she provokes.

A. Most nurses do not receive much training regarding psychological defense mechanisms; thus, this situation does not reflect on their professionalism.

B. Refusing emergency treatment would be inappropriate and would violate federal EMTALA regulations.

C. & E. These more elaborate options might be appropriate if the dispute still continued after full education regarding the psychological dynamics of the patient and advice on how to manage transference and countertransference.

ANSWER 77

A. Good sleep hygiene includes following a regular sleep schedule, maintaining a bedtime routine and a proper sleep environment, and using the bedroom primarily as a place for sleep. Regular exercise, relaxation strategies such as a warm bath, and avoiding any substances that interfere with sleep are important as well. Daytime napping may delay the expected return to sleep later that night, disrupting many of these beneficial patterns.

ANSWER 78

ANSWER 78A

I. Anorexia. Beyond an expected weight loss of at least 15% below baseline, there are several associated physical features and medical complications. Psychological features include an intense fear of gaining weight, a distorted body image, and denial of the seriousness of the illness.

ANSWER 78B

B. Delirium. The term delirium refers to a cognitive disturbance, typically of an abrupt onset with a variety of fluctuating symptoms. Reduced consciousness may differentiate this syndrome from dementia.

ANSWER 78C

F. Panic disorder. A panic attack is typically a discrete episode developing abruptly. Associated features include accelerated heart rate, derealization, and a sense of impending doom. The presence or absence of agoraphobia should also be pursued diagnostically.

ANSWER 78D

A. Major depressive episode. This disorder typically has a constellation of psychological and physical symptoms present for at least two weeks. These include feeling sad or anhedonia; worthlessness, guilt, or hopelessness; morbid thoughts; diminished concentration; appetite and sleep changes; and changes in energy level.

ANSWER 78E

C. Schizophrenia. A common evolution of this illness is gradual withdrawal and preoccupation with abstract ideas and suspiciousness. The prevalent denial of anything wrong often prevents the schizophrenic from seeking or complying with treatment.

ANSWER 78F

E. Bipolar disorder. Every patient suspected of a clinical depression should be asked about manic or hypomanic symptoms in the past to differentiate major depressive disorder from a bipolar disorder. The absence of marked grandiosity, need for hospitalization, or psychosis when manic suggests a bipolar II disorder.

ANSWER 78G

J. Bulimia. This syndrome is marked by recurrent bouts of binge eating and inappropriate compensatory behavior such as vomiting, misuse of laxatives and diuretics, fasting, or excessive exercise. A history of anorexia nervosa is not uncommon.

ANSWER 78H

G. Obsessive-compulsive disorder. Obsessions (recurrent and persistent thoughts or impulses) and compulsions (repetitive behaviors or mental acts) are hallmarks of OCD. They are perceived as excessive or unreasonable, cause marked distress, and are time-consuming.

ANSWER 78I

D. Delusional disorder. This disorder typically occurs later in life than schizophrenia and is differentiated from that condition by a lack of other psychotic symptoms. Specific delusional disorders include erotomania, jealous, grandiose, somatic, and persecutory types. Distinguishing a persecutory delusional disorder from a paranoid personality may be difficult, but expectedly the latter is longstanding.

ANSWER 78J

H. Generalized anxiety disorder. This disorder tends to be longstanding and waxes and wanes in severity. The effects of drugs, medications, or other illnesses need to be ruled out. The lack of a specific focus for the anxiety helps differentiate this condition from panic attacks, social phobia, OCD, somatization disorder, or PTSD.

ANSWER 79

B. Schizoid personality disorder is associated with behaviors of withdrawal and seeking isolation and privacy. A dependent personality disorder is unusually submissive, clinging, and indecisive with a childlike need to be taken care of by others.

ANSWER 80

ANSWER 80A

E. Adverse side effects from lithium are not uncommon even at therapeutic levels. Serious toxicity can occur at levels over 1.5 mEq/L and include altered sensorium, slurred speech, and hyperactive reflexes.

ANSWER 80B

A. Anticholinergic, antihistaminic, and adrenergic mechanisms cause a variety of physical side effects with this class of medications.

ANSWER 80C

B. These newer antidepressants are typically less bothersome than the tricyclics but are not without side effects. Sexual dysfunctions may occur in as many as 40% of patients receiving SSRIs.

ANSWER 80D

D. Although safe and effective in treating a variety of anxiety disorders, caution should be advised due to motor impairment, memory difficulties, and the potential for dependence.

ANSWER 80E

C. Adverse physical effects of this class of psychotropics are associated with their anticholinergic, antidopaminergic and antihistaminic, and alpha-adrenergic blocking properties.

ANSWER 81

E. Antipsychotics. The blockade of dopamine and other monoamine neurotransmission in the pathways that regulate thermal and neuromuscular homeostasis is associated with the neuroleptic malignant syndrome (NMS). Other signs and symptoms of NMS include diaphoresis, dysphagia, tremor, incontinence, mutism, tachycardia, leukocytosis, and laboratory evidence of muscle injury resulting in an elevated CPK.

ANSWER 82

E. Valproic acid has no particular use in the treatment of NMS. Dantrolene blocks the release of calcium from the sarcoplasmic reticulum, producing muscle relaxation. Of course, the offending antipsychotic should be stopped. Bromocriptine acts as a dopamine receptor agonist, and amantadine enhances the synthesis, release, and reuptake of dopamine. Symptomatic treatment of fever, correcting electrolyte imbalance, and managing any cardiovascular instability are necessary as well. Some studies indicate a mortality rate of nearly 12% for NMS.

ANSWER 83

E. Tardive dyskinesia is a common side effect to prolonged antipsychotic medication usage. More advanced cases may exhibit choreoathetoid movements of the limbs and trunk.

ANSWER 84

B. Males can develop tardive dyskinesia, but females have a higher risk of developing this condition. Both the prevalence and severity of TD increase with age. Unipolar depression as well as positive family history of affective disorder in relatives of schizophrenic patients are predisposing factors.

ANSWER 85

D. Haloperidol may mask the dyskinetic movements associated with TD, but ultimately this relatively pure D2 blocking agent will worsen the condition. There is no universally effective treatment for TD, but the atypical antipsychotic clozapine with serotonergic and D4 affinities has been helpful for some individuals with TD. Some patients who have had TD for a short duration benefit from the antioxidant vitamin E. Propranolol as a beta blocking agent and tetrabenazine as a monoamine depleting agent have been helpful.

ANSWER 86

A. Various twin studies have calculated concordance rates greater than 80% in monozygotic twins. This indicates non-shared or environmental factors play a role as the concordance rate is not 100%. Nonetheless genetics have become increasingly implicated in the etiology of the disease.

ANSWER 87

B. Compulsions are the best differentiating symptoms within the anxiety disorders category to make the diagnosis of OCD. Phobias and of course obsessions are common aspects of OCD. The phobias in OCD tend to become generalized over time. Obsessional ruminations are seen to some extent within all the anxiety disorders.

ANSWER 88

C. The selective serotonin reuptake inhibitors (SSRIs) are the first-line pharmacologic agents used to treat OCD. This class includes the tricyclic clomipramine as well as the more specific SSRIs such as fluoxetine, paroxetine, citalopram, sertraline, and fluvoxamine. The consulting psychiatrist suggests this patient receive fluoxetine at a starting dose of 20 mg each day.

ANSWER 89

D. Extrapyramidal symptoms are rarely seen with SSRIs. Many of the side effects associated with SSRIs are similar to those experienced with the older tricyclic antidepressants but typically not so severe.

ANSWER 90

A. Cognitive-behavioral therapy (CBT) is a helpful adjunct to pharmacotherapy of OCD. Some studies show that the long-term gains achieved with CBT exceed and are more durable than SSRIs alone.

ANSWER 91

91A. Correct Answer: D. 39%

91B. Correct Answer: C. 1%

91C. Correct Answer: B. 8%

91D. Correct Answer: E. 12%

91E. Correct Answer: A. 47%

Genetics alone are not sufficient to ensure the development of schizophrenia. Most studies imply polygenic and epigenetic contributions.

ANSWER 92

D. Mini-Mental State Exam. Answers A, B, C, and E are time-consuming and except for choice B not directly pertinent in screening for memory or cognitive deficits.

ANSWER 93

E. While each possible choice listed is assessed during the Mini-Mental State Exam, the specific request to copy the given design screens for visual-motor integrity. A correct response includes correctly copying all ten angles, two of which must intersect. The correct response is awarded a score of 1 point on this 30-point screening exam.

ANSWER 94

E. Mania. Comorbid psychiatric conditions exist in the majority of patients with panic disorders. The most frequent is agoraphobia. Depression may precede or follow the onset of a panic disorder, but mania or bipolar disorder has no particular association. A variety of "cluster C" personality disorders, including avoidant, dependent, and obsessive-compulsive personality, are associated with panic disorder. A variety of drugs, including stimulants, can precipitate a panic episode.

ANSWER 95

E. All of the above. Each of the named substances can be panicogenic in a vulnerable individual. Serotonin reuptake inhibitors and benzodiazepines have an antipanic effect. Treatment with beta-blockers does not alleviate the attacks.

ANSWER 96

D. Haloperidol is an antipsychotic with dopamine antagonist properties. Paroxetine and amitryptyline are both serotonergic agents very helpful in preventing panic episodes, as is the potent benzodiazepine alprazolam. The patients should abstain from stimulants like caffeine.

ANSWER 97

A. The withdrawal syndrome may occur any time after the blood alcohol level begins to fall.

ANSWER 98

E. Benzodiazepines are the mainstay of the treatment for alcohol withdrawal. This patient's impaired liver functioning requires a shorter-acting agent such as lorazepam or oxazepam.

ANSWER 99

B. Visual hallucinations are more common than auditory hallucinations. Auditory hallucinations can be prolonged and disturbing, sometimes lasting months and not particularly responsive to antipsychotic medications.

ANSWER 100

ANSWER 100A

C. Frontal lobe trauma results in a "frontal lobe syndrome" with associated disinhibition, apathy, and decreased curiosity.

ANSWER 100B

A. Temporal lobe damage produces loss of memory, temporal lobe epilepsy, speech disorder, and receptive and nominal dysphasia.

ANSWER 100C

D. Occipital lobe trauma causes visual field defects, color agnosia, and visual-spatial agnosia.

ANSWER 100D

B. Parietal lobe trauma can result in a variety of neuropsychiatric deficits and symptoms including ideomotor and ideational defects, disorders of body image, topographical disorientation, and constructional apraxia.